STOP EATING
YOUR HEART OUT

The 21-Day Program to Free
Yourself from Emotional Eating

MERYL HERSHEY BECK, MA, MEd, LPCC

Foreword by JEANNE RUST, PhD,
CEO/Founder, Mirasol Eating Disorder Recovery Centers

Praise for *Stop Eating Your Heart Out*

"Meryl Beck integrates some of the most effective weight management tools available into a 21-day plan that will empower you. You will also be able to identify with the author's personal story in ways that will be highly instructive for meeting your own challenges. We highly recommend this superb program."

—Donna Eden and David Feinstein, PhD,
co-authors of *Energy Medicine* and *Energy Medicine for Women*

"*Stop Eating Your Heart Out* is rich with powerful tools to heal overeating. If you are ready for change and want compassionate and nurturing support on your journey, this book may just be the recipe."

—Sylvia Haskvitz, author of *Eat by Choice, Not by Habit*

"From the first moment you start reading Meryl Beck's *Stop Eating Your Heart Out*, I think you'll feel like you're with one of your best friends—someone who loves you, cares for you, and really accepts you just the way you are. I did. Meryl's honest presence and simple, doable approaches fill the pages and made me feel supported and that her suggestions were going to be easy to follow and really helpful. If you've got the chains of emotional eating holding you back, Meryl will help you be free."

—Tapas Fleming, founder of Tapas Acupressure Technique®, tatlife.com

"*Stop Eating Your Heart Out* is a well thought out book that will help those with emotional eating find a path to recovery. Meryl Beck's personal story illuminates the journey and her practical step-by-step guide provide touchstones that anyone can follow to find healing from emotional overeating."

—Carolyn Coker Ross, MD, MPH,
author of *The Binge Eating and Compulsive Overeating Workbook*

"Meryl has written a wonderful book that demystifies Twelve-Step Recovery and brings the healing tools within Twelve-Step programs to us all. Her book is a valuable contribution in the field of emotional eating recovery. Readers will gain personal insight as well as practical tools for healing and living well."

—Joanna Poppink, MFT, psychotherapist, lecturer,
author of *Healing Your Hungry Heart*

"Meryl Hershey Beck has presented 21 self-help tools in her thought-provoking, beautifully written *Stop Eating Your Heart Out*. She creatively and artfully takes us along on her journey as she combines tried-and true recovery methods, such as the Twelve Steps, with new energy techniques. If you have a problem with over-indulging and using food instead of dealing with feelings, then open this book and discover for yourself that you too can achieve freedom from emotional eating."

—DR. JAMES DURLACHER, DC, AUTHOR OF *FREEDOM FROM FEAR FOREVER*

"An excellent resource. Here you will learn how to understand varieties of problems that contribute to overeating and how to sort these out. Helpful exercises at the end of each section will guide you on your path to a healthier, happier life."

—DANIEL J. BENOR, MD, ABIHM, AUTHOR OF *SEVEN MINUTES TO NATURAL PAIN RELEASE*

"Meryl Beck's *Stop Eating Your Heart Out* is a must have for anyone searching to make peace with food, weight, body image, and self-esteem because you will find that safe haven you are looking for right here. It is truly food for the soul. Meryl takes this complex and important issue that plagues millions and breaks it down into bite-size, palatable pieces that you can easily digest and lovingly weave into your everyday life. Plus, you will get the pleasure of absorbing all the soul-filled nutrients that are present on each page. I highly recommend this book. Your life will never be the same."

—BRONWYN MARMO, BESTSELLING AUTHOR OF *THE FOOD IS A LIE: THE TRUTH IS WITHIN*

STOP EATING
YOUR HEART OUT

The 21-Day Program to Free
Yourself from Emotional Eating

MERYL HERSHEY BECK, Ma, MEd, LPCC

Foreword by JEANNE RUST, PhD,
CEO/Founder, Mirasol Eating Disorder Recovery Centers

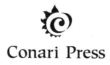

Conari Press

First published in 2011 by Conari Press, an imprint of

Red Wheel/Weiser, LLC
With offices at:
665 Third Street, Suite 400
San Francisco, CA 94107

www.redwheelweiser.com

ISBN: 978-1-57324-545-6

Library of Congress Cataloging-in-Publication Data is available upon request.

Cover design by Jim Warner
Cover image © Sandra Voogt
Interior design by ContentWorks, Inc.
Typeset in Berkeley Oldstyle

Printed in the United States of America
Malloy

10 9 8 7 6 5 4 3 2 1

The paper used in this publication meets the minimum requirements of the American National Standard for Information Sciences—Permanence of Paper for Printed Library Materials Z39.48-1992 (R1997).

In loving memory of my cherished son,
who was so proud of his mama!

Jonathan Hershey Beck
1976–2011

Contents

Foreword
· · · · · · · · · · ·

WHEN MERYL HERSHEY BECK ASKED me to write the foreword for her new book, I was ecstatic. I must tell you that I absolutely love Meryl Beck! I have treated eating disorders for nearly twenty-five years, including twelve years as the CEO of Mirasol, an integrative eating-disorder treatment program. During that time, I've had the pleasure of working with Meryl and sharing a common interest in energy psychology.

When I'm with Meryl, the room is full of light. And now Meryl has written a book that illuminates the true path to recovery from compulsive eating. She is a recovered individual who has survived the ups and downs of living life on life's terms and has survived the emotional journey of those who seek that often elusive true path to healing.

Every morning millions of people get up, go into the bathroom, and say, "Good morning, Mr. Scale." Mr. Scale is the one who determines if they're going to have a good day or a bad day. Bad scale days are damaging to self-esteem and emotional well-being. Billions of dollars are spent in the diet industry every year, yet people are continuing to get fatter.

This last year alone, obesity rates rose in seventeen states, and obesity is now contributing to most of our healthcare costs. Currently one-third of all Americans are obese, one-third are overweight, and the rest are of a normal and healthy weight. The majority of the people in this country are told they should lose some weight. This includes not only adults but, sadly, children and babies as well.

I remember growing up in an overweight family that was always on a diet. I remember when my parents would come home from the grocery store, all smiles as they brought in the grocery bags. All of a sudden, everything in life was wonderful. We all breathed a sigh of relief because we had an abundance of food in the house. Happiness in my house was a full refrigerator. When my mother died, my brother and I walked through her home and found four refrigerators and three freezers, all full. Both of my parents were heavy and died relatively early deaths due to heart disease. Of course, what they really died of was compulsive eating.

There are many books about binge eating, but few are written with the openness, clarity, and authenticity of *Stop Eating Your Heart Out*. Meryl begins with a quiz to help you determine whether or not you have a problem. Then, ever so gently, she leads you into a provocative twenty-one-day program that teaches the difference between food and feelings. The focus of the program is not about weight loss but about learning to recognize when you're engaging in emotional eating, which Meryl believes is at the core of a binge eating disorder.

Most experts agree that eating disorders are caused by a combination of biogenetic, psychological, and socio-cultural factors. Meryl teaches us how to live in recovery. No matter what caused the disorder, what matters now is finding peace with our bodies, forming new identities, and becoming acquainted with our true selves.

Stop Eating Your Heart Out provides a step-by-step path to wellness using strategies that are designed for the real world. Humorous anecdotes sprinkled with wisdom and informational insights help add new dimensions to our thinking.

I would suggest that you read the book a little at a time—as you would savor a good meal—and slowly begin to integrate Meryl's suggestions. Whether you're living in recovery or just beginning the journey, this wonderful book will add tremendously to your knowledge. You'll see why I love Meryl Beck! And why I love the path to recovery she has chosen.

—Jeanne Rust, PhD
CEO and Founder,
Mirasol Eating Disorder Treatment Centers
Tucson, Arizona

Acknowledgments
. . . .

*Let us be grateful to people who make us happy; they are
the charming gardeners who make our souls blossom.*

—Marcel Proust, *Pleasure and Days*

I AM VERY APPRECIATIVE OF the many individuals and "family" groups who have made my soul bloom throughout my journey.

My biological family was with me through thick and thin, literally. Although I had challenges growing up, my parents, May and Bob Hershey, always did the best they could and I feel incredibly loved by them. I can also always count on my sister and brother, Bonnie and Denny Hershey; family love runs strong through our veins and hearts!

My illustrator, the talented, wise, generous, and very loving Alison Hershey Manes is also my beloved daughter. She is a blessing in my life, as are her five awesome daughters who bring me immense joy.

The Twelve-Step Recovery community became my family of choice in the 1970s and gave me the best education I ever received (and I have two master degrees!). These folks loved me until I learned to love myself and I am forever grateful. With their help and support, I experienced physical, emotional, mental, and spiritual recovery: I learned about feelings, had a spiritual awakening, began to engage in healthy eating, and moved into self-acceptance.

My spiritual family also loves me unconditionally, and I am very thankful for them. Robin Trainor Masci, my best friend, was the first person to hold up a mirror and show me the awesomeness of my true self; I am immensely grateful that I can always count on her friendship and her love. Many others have been my cheerleaders and supporters as I wrote this book, including Janet Mooney, who makes me laugh every day and strongly encourages the best in me; Mark Naseck, my soul brother, who celebrates all the victories with me, and Glenn Richards, my first "groupie." I am appreciative of many others, way too numerous to mention, who hold the energy for me and see me in my highest self.

An acknowledgment also goes to my writing family. In 2009 I attended Tom Bird's writing retreat and birthed this book. I am grateful for Tom's encouragement and for the support of all my classmates, especially my roommate, Jerelyn Schultz, and the Tucson writing group that was formed with Mimi Villifane, CJ Walker, Jan, and Jere.

Many folks worked with me in the revision stage of the book. Thanks to Laura George for her reassurance and care in helping me through the writing-publishing process. Mary Langford did a phenomenal job assisting with the submission package and the first few chapters of the book before she became ill; working with her was easy and fun, and I continue to pray for her optimal health. When I needed quick editing help, Mimi and Ellie Starer graciously jumped in. Then the very observant eyes of Andra Ewton and Windy Jones took over and I relished being able to count on them, the ease of working with them, and the invaluable suggestions they made.

Conari Press has become my newest family, and I am so thankful that my dear friend Nancy Burson recommended them. I feel indebted to Caroline Pincus who told me my writing was "terrific. Just terrific," and decided to take a chance on me, an unknown author. The editorial help I have received from Caroline Pincus and Susie Pitzen has been invaluable and I look forward to working with Martha Knauf and Pat Rose and everyone else at Conari who is going to bat for me (and the book)!

Jeanne Rust has been a friend for several years and I so appreciate her believing in me, seeing my light, and writing the foreword.

Although I don't always get to the conferences, the energy psychology community has felt like a family to me and holds a special place in my heart. We are all indebted to Kate Sorenson, my incredibly wise soul sister, who instituted the Energy Psychology Conference in 1999, and to my ingenious teacher and colleague, Gary Craig, who so generously gave EFT (Emotional Freedom Techniques) to the world.

And finally, I applaud my clients and the many women I sponsored for trusting me enough to test out the methods discussed throughout this book. It has been a blessing to walk beside them and support them in their growth and recovery.

Thank you.

Introduction

· · · · · · · · · · · · · ·

Not everything that is faced can be changed, but
nothing can be changed until it is faced.
—JAMES BALDWIN, *THE CROSS OF REDEMPTION: UNCOLLECTED WRITINGS*

DESPITE THE FACT THAT AMERICANS are obsessed with weight and spend over $60 billion a year on diets and diet products, has it done any good?

The media screams out to us on a daily basis: *We have an obesity epidemic!* According to the Center for Disease Control and Prevention, over two-thirds of Americans are overweight or obese. Many of the millions of heavy people have an eating disorder, which has the highest mortality rate of any mental health diagnosis, including depression. Binge eating, the most common eating disorder in the United States, affects over twenty-five million people. This diagnosis has received a lot of media attention recently because the American Psychiatric Association is recommending that it be considered a separate, distinct eating disorder, as are bulimia and anorexia.

Though not all obese individuals are compulsive overeaters, experts believe that about 75 percent of overeating is emotional eating—using food to deal with feelings. Although everyone turns to food for comfort on occasion, such as hot soup or hot chocolate on a cold winter's night, or something sweet to chew on after a fight with your honey, the compulsive overeater turns to food as the primary means of coping with everyday stress, anxiety, and other difficult feelings. We have an emotional hunger. Some of us eat because of an inner emptiness, and some of us become addicted to sugar and refined carbohydrates as a result. "Fast food has become the opiate of the masses," fitness trainer Chris Powell declared on *Extreme Makeover: Weight Loss Edition.* Compulsive eating begins as an attempt to ease emotional pain, but it ends up making us feel even worse.

As a licensed professional clinical counselor, I have worked with compulsive overeaters and binge eaters for over twenty years. In addition, I, too, am a (recovered) food junkie and spent many years quelling feelings by shoving ice cream or cookies down my throat. Food was the glue that kept me together.

Some folks with excess weight just eat a bit too much. Emotional eaters like me, however, use food as a fix: I abused food, just as an alcoholic misuses booze, stuffing myself in an attempt to fill an inner emptiness. For many of us, though, there is not enough food on the planet to fill the gaping hole within our souls. I know—I tried.

During my compulsive overeating days, I spent my time bingeing; hoarding and hiding food; making food my best friend; sneak eating; taking pills to curb my appetite; going to diet doctors; gaining and losing a gazillion pounds; trying different fad diets; hating myself; loathing my body; making and breaking countless self-promises; and feeling helpless and hopeless. I ate frozen food that tasted like cardboard; I finished the food off my children's plates; I retrieved food that had been thrown away; I confiscated my students' candy and ate it myself. I expressed lots of dishonesty around food, masquerading as the supreme dieter in public and experiencing out-of-control bingeing in private.

My behavior around food was a closely guarded secret for decades. But not anymore. After years of psychotherapy, working the Twelve Steps, and doing focused personal-growth work, I have gained insight and understanding as to why I became an emotional eater at an early age and why compulsive overeating became such a driving force in my life. Fortunately, I have recovered from my binge eating disorder, and the tools I used are presented here. I share my journey candidly so that others may benefit from my experiences.

Tools

As I disclose my ordeals with food and out-of-control eating, I am telling the story of millions of others who use food to self-soothe. With the focus on recovery, however, I share the modalities that worked for me, including the spiritual approach I first encountered in support groups using Twelve-Step Recovery. No one method will work for every person, and rest assured that successful use of this book does not depend on adherence to a Twelve-Step Program. I didn't adapt the Alcoholics Anonymous program to my food issues by myself—it's served as a model for many over the years. Overeaters Anonymous (OA), for instance, began in 1960 and uses the same Twelve Steps as AA, substituting the word *food* for *alcohol*. It is open to anyone with issues around food, including those with binge eating disorder, bulimia, and anorexia. Other Twelve-Step groups dealing with food issues include Food Addicts Anonymous (FAA), Eating Addictions Anonymous (EAA), Food Addicts in Recovery Anonymous (FA), and Eating Disorders Anonymous (EDA). These, plus more, are listed in the back of the book under Resources.

Although many people, including me, have achieved remarkable recovery with the help of a Twelve-Step support group, I know that some of you are not drawn to that approach. And that's perfectly okay. This book introduces you to a range of wonderfully effective self-help tools, such as Inner Child work, creative visualizations, journaling, and various energy techniques that together can help you rewire your brain to stop craving food.

In my own work as a teacher and psychotherapist, I use some approaches that fall under the umbrella of energy psychology. Based in Eastern medicine, energy psychology is sometimes described as needleless acupuncture. It is a relatively new term to describe various modalities or approaches that use the body's energy systems to create change for the individual. Many energy psychology techniques employ repeating an affirmation while tapping or touching acupressure points to release unpleasant emotions or to eliminate cravings. These techniques are highly effective at diminishing anxiety and other uncomfortable feelings that send many of us directly to the cookie jar. In fact, without also working on the body's energy system, thinking and reason alone rarely work.

Using This Book

I recommend keeping a computer or notebook nearby while you read. Though you're of course free to mark up the margins as much as you like, this book isn't meant to be a workbook, so there's not much blank space.

The bulk of this book is devoted to my twenty-one-day program for releasing you from your emotional dependence on food, but first I want to tell you my own story. You'll find that in chapter 1. Each subsequent chapter (except the last) covers three days, with a new tool introduced each day to add to your own toolbox. You might choose to do an assignment in a day, or you might want to take a whole week to do one. That's entirely up to you. Of course, if you take more than a day, the process outlined here will take more than twenty-one days. But once you have completed all the assignments, you will have all the tools you need to recover from emotional eating. These are tools that you can use over and over again or just once. However you need them to work, they will. The final chapter of the program, Conscious Living, discusses ways to keep using the contents of your personal toolbox as you continue to forge your new life, free from emotional eating.

For many years, I thought I was terminally unique. But the more I shared myself, the more I realized that others had the same thoughts, the same actions, and the same beliefs I did. If you are anything like I was, you've been waiting a long time to conquer your battle with food and self-hatred.

You're not alone. Begin this next phase of your journey by turning the pages and encountering many new techniques. Please try them all, and then pick and choose the ones you find most useful to create your own individualized toolbox. In so doing, you will alleviate the compulsive overeating as you transform yourself and your relationship to food. In the words of English novelist and critic Aldous Huxley, "There is only one corner of the universe you can be certain of improving, and that's your own self."

Chapter 1

My Story: The Making and Breaking of a Compulsive Overeater

. . . .

We must go beyond our history to arrive at our destiny.
—ALAN COHEN, *DARE TO BE YOURSELF*

"SEE THOSE FAT PEOPLE OVER there?" my father asked as we drove down the street, his finger pointing at a group of overweight people.

"Yes, Daddy," I replied.

"You don't ever want to look like that!" he admonished.

I was an impressionable eight-year-old girl. It was the 1950s, a time when looking good mattered most. World War II had ended the previous decade, and with no external war to contend with, many families like ours focused on social appearance and physical attractiveness. Airlines had stewardesses, not flight attendants, who were obligated to conform to specific weight, height, and age requirements. They had to look good to keep their jobs. This was the time of *Leave It to Beaver* and *Father Knows Best*—those happy TV families with the pearl-wearing housewives decked out in heels, even at breakfast. I was part of a looking-good family in a looking-good culture, most of us holding the belief that in order to be accepted, we must look acceptable. And, having weight issues ever since I was a little kid, I felt like the ugly duckling of the family.

Children like to please their parents; the praise it evokes feels good. I made my parents very happy by being an amiable and obedient child. And, as a charter member of the Clean Plate Club, I was commended at mealtime for eating and finishing all the food in front of me—beginning when I was a baby in a highchair. The conditioning had begun.

Always eager to do what was expected of me, I was mortified when, as a three-year-old, I misunderstood my parents and felt humiliation for the first time: My mother walked into the living room and saw my feet thrust into the playpen, which also contained my baby sister. When my mother asked what I was doing, I calmly replied that she had said I could touch only the baby's feet, so I was letting my sister touch mine. It made perfect sense to me, but hearing the thunderous roar of laughter spewing forth from the adults as she immediately recounted the story, I was mortified. At the tender age of three, I made a decision to never make a mistake again—the shame was too great and I felt crushed.

I set out to be "the best little girl in the world"—to be perfect and do everything right. Inside I felt very alone—a feeling heightened by my father traveling a lot for business and my mother being emotionally unavailable. It wasn't long before I discovered that stuffing myself with food was a great way to take the edge off the emptiness inside.

When I was six, my brother was born, and the hoopla surrounding the birth of a male said to me that boys matter and girls don't. I felt negated for being "just a girl." The hole inside me continued to grow, and I bolted through meals in an attempt to fill the void. I was losing the ability to feel physical hunger—I ate to feel full and to numb out. I ate large portions whenever possible. I ate with gusto, and I wanted to feel stuffed.

Although never diagnosed, I exhibited many of the symptoms of childhood depression. I had very little energy; many times on my walk home from school I had to push myself to take the next step and then the next. I felt depressed about my weight and disgrace around it. Life was not fun; it was an ordeal to be lived through. No, life was an ordeal to be *smiled* through. Smile, no matter what I am feeling. Smile, no matter what is happening. Smile, to keep my inner pain a secret.

As I grew older, I became more and more quiet and isolated. A voracious reader, I kept to myself most of the time with my nose in a book. In the presence of others, I did whatever I was expected to do—filling the role of the good student, the good helper, the good daughter, and the good sister. I put on my *I am wonderful* mask, wore a smile on my face, and suppressed my feelings. Even though I often acted like the hero of the family, I usually felt like the invisible lost child. I needed extra food to pull this off.

I first realized my dissatisfaction with my body during my preteen years. When I was seated, a roll of fat protruded around my belly. One day my father grabbed it and said in a teasing voice, "What's *this?*" I felt humiliated. I had something on my body that wasn't accepted, and I couldn't hide the fat. My body image issues had begun.

I knew I needed to lose weight, and the next morning I wrote in my diary: "Today I am starting my diet." The following day I wrote: "Yesterday I had a chocolate-chip cookie. Today I am *really* starting my diet." Then the next day I scribbled: "Yesterday I had some candy. Today I *am really, really starting my diet!*"

Each day I would pledge to start again. For me, in those days, dieting meant I wouldn't have any sweets, and it was a struggle to not eat sugar. Visiting a friend's house, I'd often sneak into the kitchen and surreptitiously wolf down cookies or chocolate chip-muffins. Or I found excuses to go to my next-door neighbor's house, where, when no one was looking, I'd head straight for the candy drawer, which was always filled with chocolate haystacks and other mouth-watering goodies.

Although the portions were substantial at our family meals, I always wanted more so I would feel satiated. When I'd ask for another helping, Mom or Dad might remark, "Didn't you have enough?" or, more emphatically, "You've had plenty!" The only way I could consume enough to feel full was to eat in secret, and early on I developed my talent for sneaking food to not feel so empty. For example, my mother would sometimes bring home a loaf of fresh, warm, Jewish rye bread, and I'd creep into the kitchen and snatch slices from the middle, pushing the ends closer together so it just looked like a smaller loaf. I'd gobble the bread down as fast as I could—without ever tasting it—so nobody would see me.

When I was ten, I entered a pancake-eating contest and easily won. And I could have kept on eating—I only stopped cramming in the pancakes because they had already named me the winner. I liked those eating contests. They were the only times I would allow others to see how much I could consume.

Somehow I fooled everyone about my eating behavior, and no one seemed to know the quantity I consumed. It was important for me to eat in secret because criticism shattered me. Jarring words cut into me like a scathing sword. I chose to be good and look good to avoid harsh judgments and disapproval. At one point, I even wished I had a tapeworm. I thought it would be the perfect solution—scarf down as much food as I wanted and let the tapeworm eat it so I wouldn't gain weight. I also considered swallowing Mexican jumping beans—maybe the larva inside each bean would consume my fat!

When I look back at early childhood photos, I don't see a grossly fat kid. Yes, sometimes a little chunky, but not obese. My parents, however, believed I needed to lose weight, and the diets began at age eleven. They took me to the family doctor, who put me on my first diet and gave me a shot once a week. I became stoic, rolled up my sleeve for the injection, and never complained. Although I kept my feelings submerged, I still felt them. I believed I was inferior and defective—land mines for compulsive overeaters like me. And, though I lost weight, I was never able to keep it off.

As a teen, I identified with the lyrics of a popular Platters song, "The Great Pretender"—pretending to do well but really feeling very alone. I saw myself as an impostor. Every day in seventh grade I'd walk home from school with classmates, and we'd always cut through the local department store. Meandering through the Juniors department, the other girls looked at the size 5 and 7 clothing. I feigned looking at the size 9s and 11s, as if I wore that size. Who was I fooling? I was squeezing myself into a size 15.

Yes, I pretended a lot. I pretended it didn't matter to me that my daddy was gone all week and I felt abandoned. I pretended I didn't care if no one gave me a compliment or if I wasn't asked out on a date. I got so used to pretending that I lost track of what was real and what was the world I invented or pretended to live in.

Since I had mastered the art of closet eating, I knew I was tricking others into believing I was constantly on a diet and ate only low-calorie food. When eating out with friends, I'd order a small meal and never anything fattening. But I had to eat something substantial beforehand in order to pull off this charade. If I had consumed solely what I allowed others to see me eating, I probably would have weighed 90 pounds!

But I didn't weigh 90 pounds, and I had a strong reaction to the numbers on the scale. If the scale read 125–130, my spirits were high and I loved life. When the scale read 150, I hated myself, verbally lambasted myself, and everything looked dark and bleak. It perplexed me how my weight fluctuated 25 pounds—it felt as if I'd get up one day and the numbers on the scale had mysteriously jumped way up.

As teenagers, my friends began dating, but I spent my Saturday nights babysitting—a job I loved. I was in compulsive-overeater heaven: unlimited use of the phone, my favorite TV shows, and snacks galore. I convinced myself it didn't matter that I didn't date; I had my babysitting job, so I was alone with my real love: the food!

I tried "diet pills," which I found out later were speed. But instead of feeling wired, I felt extremely tired. Several of my friends loved these new pills and seemed to get skinnier by the minute. Once again I felt defective. Why did these pills work for others but not for me? What was *wrong* with me?

During a routine physical, I was diagnosed with an underactive thyroid. I heard this with great excitement and hope—thyroid medication was, I thought, the magic pill I had been looking for. Now the weight would fall off. No such luck—I took the thyroid meds, but the weight hung on.

I was continually on the lookout for the latest diet craze and was filled with high expectations when I discovered Metrecal—the first diet drink. Used as a meal replacement (except by my grandmother, who misunderstood and drank it with her meals and then wondered why she didn't lose weight!), I drank it for lunch each day. But I didn't achieve the much-desired weight loss. I tried fad diets and other diet pills. I chewed on AYDS (an appetite suppressant tasting so much like chocolate candy that I ate many more than the recommended one piece). I went to Diet Workshop. I followed the Weight Watchers diet. Sometimes I lost weight, but if it was lost, it was soon found. I felt disappointed and hopeless about the numbers on the scale. The immensity of these feelings increased my appetite, and I'd pig out even more.

There were times when I tried to be bulimic—in part to lose weight and in part to relieve indigestion—and, thank goodness, I was not successful. Although I'd put my fingers down my throat, I was not able to regurgitate the large volume of food I had consumed. Instead, antacids became my trusted ally, eventually easing the horrendous pain in my gut from gorging.

At an early age, I lost my sense of self and became more interested in what others felt or needed. I thought of myself as a chameleon—you tell me who you want me to be, and I'll be it. As long as others were happy, my needs were inconsequential. (It sounds like initiation for martyrdom.) I negated my own feelings, pushed them down, and gave them no importance. Out of touch with myself, I didn't know how I felt most of the time. I was conditioned to put on a happy front no matter what happened. To keep up this charade, I was compelled to consume an enormous amount of food.

I felt a lot of guilt and shame. The shame intensified when I received critical comments from my parents such as "You're the oldest—why would you even ask such a question?" or "You know better than that!" or "Why did you do that? What kind of example are you setting?" I became hypervigilant—seeking to anticipate my parents' every need rather than be reprimanded. It wasn't enough, however, because their voices took residence in my head, and I used those messages to rebuke myself, often by calling myself stupid. Is it any wonder I turned to food for love? To feel full? No, actually, to *not* feel.

As a high school English teacher, I taught the poem "Richard Cory" by Edwin Arlington Robinson. Richard Cory seemed to have it all—he had money, he had friends, people admired him and wished they could be him. I thought my life sounded a lot like Richard Cory's: People liked me and respected me and thought I was very responsible—an image I had worked hard to create. But Richard Cory went home one night and put a bullet through his head—and I understood. I realized the outward appearance might just be a cover-up; I knew his pain. On the outside I had everything—a nice home, a hardworking husband, two cars in our garage, enough money, plenty of food. Yet inside I was tormented. I told myself over and over that I was inadequate and defective, and that I was a fraud.

I knew I was a sneak eater, and I knew I ate to the point of physical distress, but I didn't know until recently that I had a binge eating disorder. The mental health description of *binge eating disorder* includes the following:

1. Eating a large amount of food in a short period of time
2. Lack of control over eating during the binge episode
3. Eating until uncomfortably full

4. Eating large amounts of food when not physically hungry

5. Eating much more rapidly than normal

6. Eating alone because you are embarrassed by how much you're eating

7. Feeling disgusted, depressed, or guilty after overeating

I easily identified with each aspect:

1. Yes, I could pack it away.

2. In the midst of a binge, I would command my hand to stop shoving cookies into my mouth, but it wouldn't stop.

3. I would eat so much that my stomach ached intensely. I'd chew a few Pepto-Bismol tablets and curl up in the fetal position until the pain sub-sided—and then I'd get up and feast some more.

4. I know I ate because of emotional, not physical, hunger.

5. I inhaled my food.

6. I always preferred eating alone so I wouldn't be judged.

7. Disgusted, depressed, or guilty? Yes, yes, and yes! I was often all three. That's why I became a closet eater in the first place.

When I was twenty-nine, a friend told me she had attended a Twelve-Step meeting for people with weight issues. "There really is a place like that?" I asked incredulously. Many years earlier, as a child, I had seen the teleplay *Days of Wine and Roses,* which depicts the total devastation of an alcoholic's life before he achieves sobriety with the help of Alcoholics Anonymous. At that time, I thought, "Wow, I wish there was a place like that for me—I'm a *foodaholic.*" That's what I'd called myself since the age of twelve. I knew that whenever I started to eat, I didn't want to stop. I had to contain myself or get scolded for eating too much. I knew I had an emptiness no amount of food would fill. Actually, I didn't know that then. But I know it now. Thinking back, I wonder if my appestat (the area of the brain that controls the appetite) was broken.

I accompanied my friend to the next Twelve-Step support group and, right away, made a decision to follow the 3-0-1 food plan: three meals a day, nothing in between, one day at a time. What a struggle. It was almost impossible for me to refrain from eating between meals. Whenever I drove past my favorite bakery, for example, my car would automatically turn in. At the beginning, over and over again I fell off the wagon, which is how I saw it in my mind. As I continued going to meetings and working the Twelve Steps, I began to get truthful with myself about my feelings and started to let go of the ludicrous notion that I had to be flawless. And, lo and behold, the emotional eating began to wane. When, months later, I drove past the bakery and didn't stop, I was elated. After that first success came many more, and soon I could drive past all bakeries without pulling in.

Committed to not eating between meals, I developed a technique to delay immediate gratification: If I really wanted a particular food, if something "called" to me, I gave myself permission to have it—tomorrow, and with a meal. For instance, if my husband decided to eat popcorn in the evening while we watched TV and I wanted it, too, I told myself I could have it . . . with a meal . . . tomorrow. And that worked for me. Sometimes I devoured that coveted food with my very next meal (such as popcorn for breakfast!). But at least it was planned for my meal, rather than a binge. Often, though, since I didn't immediately act on the craving, the obsession went away and I forgot all about it.

As a member of a Twelve-Step Program (and following a specific food plan), I eventually stopped the emotional eating by

- strengthening my spirituality (a belief in a Higher Power who loves me unconditionally),
- becoming honest with myself,
- facing my feelings,
- having a support group,
- admitting my faults,
- making amends,
- journaling,
- healing my Inner Child,
- calming my Inner Critic's voice,
- white-knuckling it.

My eating behavior now is a far cry from my eating behavior as a child, teen, and young woman, when I was using food as my "fix." Food used to be my best friend, my savior, my everything. Now food is just food. I enjoy it much more today than when I was rapidly shoveling it in without stopping to savor a single bite.

Twelve-Step Recovery was my first undertaking in finding myself. I entered those support-group rooms a shame-based woman with low self-esteem, but I presented myself as better than everyone to cover up the inferiority I felt. I had a deep inner desire to let others know who I really was—but I was terrified that when they found out who I truly was, I would be rejected. Taking the risk, I began to disclose myself a little at a time, chipping away at the wall I had constructed. As I came out of hiding, love and compassion were reflected back to me. I no longer felt alone. I had a sense of belonging, and the Twelve-Step fellowships became my family of choice.

Being a sponsor for many women in Twelve-Step Recovery, and going to therapy myself, paved the way for me to make a career change in 1990. I obtained a master's degree in counseling and became a psychotherapist. As a licensed professional clinical counselor (LPCC), I specialize in working with the Twelve-Step Recovery population, with a focus on eating disorders (mainly binge eating disorder and compulsive overeating). In the 1990s I developed and ran outpatient food abuse treatment weeks, helping clients heal their relationship with food. The participants recognized they were emotional eaters, with anxiety their biggest trigger of all. It was interesting to discover that every attendee had family members who were either alcoholic or obese. Experts agree there is a genetic component to obesity (I had two very large grandmothers) and a heavy correlation with alcoholism.

For many years, compulsive overeating beat me down until I embraced the tools for change. I have changed, thanks in large measure to a process of uncovering and accepting who I really am. Just like you, I'm not immune to distressing feelings. When I become aware of them, I go to my toolbox to deal with whatever is troubling me, rather than grabbing something to eat to push them away.

You, too, can conquer emotional eating.

Let's get started!

Chapter 2

Becoming Self-Honest

The longest journey is the journey inward, for he who has chosen his destiny has started upon his quest for the source of his being.

—DAG HAMMARSKJÖLD, MARKINGS

AS OLIVER HARDY MIGHT HAVE said to his sidekick, Stan Laurel, "This is a fine mess we've gotten ourselves into." No, they weren't referring to weight, but we certainly can apply that to us!

Emotional eating, binge eating, compulsive overeating—whatever we want to call it, the actions and results are similar: out-of-control eating often resulting in overweight or obesity. For our purposes here, the words *binge eater*, *compulsive overeater*, and *emotional eater* will be used interchangeably, as they are all meant to imply the same thing—using food to satisfy our emotional needs.

Emotional overeating involves eating large quantities of food in a short period of time, feeling out of control during these binges, eating rapidly, eating without physical hunger, choosing to eat alone, grazing (nibbling at food all day), and/or feeling depressed about overeating.

What caused us to become compulsive overeaters? Many of us grew up in homes where we lived with anxiety and found comfort in food. Many of us grew up with criticism and shame and found an escape in food. Many of us grew up believing we were imperfect and needed to hide that feeling of imperfection by stuffing our faces (or, in reality, our bellies). Here is a list that describes some of us. As you read through it, count how many apply to you all or much of the time:

- I am preoccupied with food, eating, and weight.
- I am aware that my eating patterns are not normal.
- I eat when I am not physically hungry.
- I eat very little in public and binge in private.
- I eat to comfort myself and relieve distressing feelings.
- I tend to eat more when I am stressed, anxious, or depressed.
- I graze all day, often needing something in my mouth.
- Food has become my friend, my lover, or my drug of choice.
- I sometimes feel hungry even after a large meal.
- I eat more rapidly than other people.
- I allow the scale to determine if I have a good or bad day.
- I eat until my stomach hurts or I feel nauseated.

- I feel ashamed of myself due to the quantity of food I consume.
- I feel powerless over my eating behavior.
- I eat before I go to bed at night so I can sleep.
- I use food as a reward.
- I eat when I am bored, tired, or feeling blah.
- I eat when I see food ads on TV.
- I often stop to get fast food and eat it in the car.
- I am secretive about what I eat and how much I eat.
- I eagerly anticipate the times I can eat alone.
- I am an overachiever and want to be in control.
- I often think I am worthless or not good enough.
- I frequently compare my body size to that of others.
- I make derogatory jokes about my eating or body size.
- I have tried many diets, unsuccessfully.
- I am terrified that I will keep gaining weight.

Going through the list helps you become conscious of some of your patterns around food and weight issues. If you recognize yourself in three or more, you are probably a compulsive overeater. Congratulate yourself for your truthfulness. We cannot change that which is hidden; bringing all this up and out is necessary in the process of healing and self-growth.

You might not have thought about food as a drug, but think about how you use it. Addicts and alcoholics use their drugs/alcohol to anesthetize themselves. Is that what you are doing with food? Addicts and alcoholics use their drug of choice as a mood-altering substance to escape from emotional pain. What do you use to escape your feelings? Food, right? This is not about making you feel wrong or bad. It is about shedding light on the activity you desire to change—your compulsive eating. It is about coming out of hiding and admitting to yourself that you use food just as alcoholics use booze. It is about admitting to yourself that you need your food fix just like dope addicts need their drug fix.

Take a deep breath—this may be a lot to take in. Again, being food dependent does not mean you're bad. You have a dependency, and as you read on and do the assignments, you will acquire tools to lessen the need to use and abuse food.

Day (1) Eating History

In chapter 1, I shared that my struggles with food and weight began when I was a child. What about you? As you move into this phase of your life journey, it is time for you to take a look at your history with food, diets, and weight issues. So much of our eating is unconscious that you might not be cognizant of your eating history. Do the best you can. Looking at old photos and reading old diary entries can help.

My clients often gasp when I tell them to write their eating history. When I hear the comment "Why do *you* need to know?" I explain that it is really about them getting honest with themselves and *their* need to know.

Start to think about it for yourself. Beginning with childhood, what has been your relationship with food?

Did you start compulsive overeating as a youngster? Did the binge eating start in adulthood? What were the events that led up to it?

Here are excerpts from a few of my clients' eating histories:

> As a child I was a picky eater and there were many battles at the dinner table. I wasn't allowed to leave until I ate everything on my plate, and sometimes I sat there for hours until my mom finally gave up and told me to go to bed. I didn't have trouble with food or weight until after I had kids. Then, never wanting to waste food, I always finished what they left on their plates. Interesting how I used to be picky, and now I eat anything rather than throwing it out.

> I have always liked food, and we had big family celebrations with a lot of food. Both my parents are heavy, my grandparents, too. We just like to eat a lot.

> My mom worked and I was in charge of making the family dinners starting when I was about eight. I got to be a really good cook. I love when people appreciate the food I make, and I serve big portions. I love to eat, too. But now it is out of control, I am obese, I have health problems, and I know I eat too much junk food.

> I was always a normal weight until my sister died when I was twenty. We didn't have a very good

relationship, and I felt bad that I wasn't nicer to her. After she died, food just seemed to taste better, so I ate more and more. That was twenty-five years ago, and I am still eating a lot.

I got pregnant as a teen and was ostracized by my family. Before that, food was just food. Being pregnant, they told me I was eating for two and I gained a lot of weight. I never lost my baby weight and my daughter is now twelve. I like eating rich foods like pasta with Alfredo sauce, big desserts, and lots of bread and butter.

My children are skinny, so I always have snack food around for them. But I eat it, they don't. When I know it is there, I can't stop myself. I think I am only going to have one or two cookies, and then I eat six, eight, ten, or more. I can't control myself.

I was a normal weight growing up, and then I got married. My husband loves to eat, and we go to buffets a lot. We get along the best when I am his eating buddy, and I have started to enjoy it. I did it for him, and now it feels like I am hooked and can't stop myself from overeating.

I started dieting when I was a preteen because I was pudgy. All through my teen years I was on one diet or another. I couldn't stay on any of them very long and soon I was back to my binge eating. I am now forty-eight, and I don't know how to stay on a diet, and I don't know how to lose weight. Please help me!

I grew up believing there was good food, like fruits and vegetables, and bad food, like candy and desserts. Our home hardly ever had any of the bad food, so whenever I went to someone else's house I ate as much of it as I could. I used to fill my pockets with the candy and then hide it in my room so I wouldn't get yelled at.

There wasn't any set mealtime at our house. We just ate whenever and whatever we wanted. I remember, night after night, fixing myself a box of macaroni and cheese and then eating the whole pot. I didn't have a problem with weight until I hit forty and then I suddenly gained about twenty pounds. That was twenty-five years ago—and fifty pounds ago!

Many clients, many stories. Yours may sound similar to some of these or totally different. It doesn't matter—it is your personal history with food and eating. You'll have the opportunity to begin contemplating how you've used food as you work on today's assignment.

Assignment

If you don't already have your notebook or your computer near you, get it now. Starting with details from as far back as you can remember, write your eating history. Discuss your relationship with food from childhood to the present. What was mealtime like with your family? When did you begin to have weight issues? When did the overeating/bingeing begin? What foods or food groups do you crave? How has food been your security blanket? Write in as much detail as you can, being as truthful as possible. What messages did you give yourself about your eating? What messages did others give you about your eating and your weight?

Day (2) Food–Mood Diary

Yesterday's assignment was about the past, and perhaps it gave you some aha moments. Today we move to the present as we begin to explore the connection between food and feelings, between stimulus and response.

It's not what you're eating; it's what's eating you. In my days of recovering from binge eating disorder, I heard this again and again. What was it that caused me to put food in my mouth when I was not physically hungry? I ate when I was sad, anxious, ashamed, and afraid. Whenever I had an unpleasant feeling, I wanted food to push it away, to sedate me. When I was angry, I often chose crunchy foods like potato chips. When I felt lonely, I chose sweets.

Many people are quite new to thinking about and identifying their feelings. Since I was very much out of touch with my emotions when I began recovery, I had a difficult time with this. I grew up in the 1950s in what was mostly a positive family. That might sound nice and enviable; however, there was no space for any feelings other than happy ones in such a family. At age four, I felt very sad and abandoned when my father changed jobs and became a traveling salesman. He was sometimes gone for weeks, but usually he left on Monday morning and returned Friday night. As a little girl, I expressed my feelings to my mother, and she would say, "Oh, no, honey, you don't feel sad." Or, "You shouldn't feel sad—you'll be getting new toys and presents." Or, "Here, honey, have a cookie and you'll feel better!" The message came through loud and clear: It wasn't okay to feel unhappy.

I quickly discovered that food could push away disagreeable feelings and alter my mood, and that's probably when my compulsive overeating began. Since I was so out of touch with my feelings, when I filled in any kind of food-mood chart, I often left the Feelings section blank or filled it in with the word *hungry*. *Hungry*, though, is not an emotional feeling.

When we were children, big feelings were so large and overwhelming we thought they'd kill us. Now, as adults, we might still be thinking that the big feelings will annihilate us. But they won't. They cause pain, maybe. Death, no.

Assignment

You're going to create your food-mood diary today. Write the following words across the top of a blank page:

<u>Time</u>   <u>Food</u>   <u>Feeling</u>   <u>Precipitating Event</u>

Every time you eat anything for the next twenty-one days (yes, just one bite of something counts), fill in the chart. Below is an example of a chart for one day:

<u>Time</u>	<u>Food</u>	<u>Feeling</u>	<u>Precipitating Event</u>
8:00	eggs	annoyed	I overslept.
10:00	chips	angry	My dog pooped on the floor.
Noon	chicken salad sandwich, carrots	happy	Having lunch with a friend.
2:00	Snickers bar	hurt	My meeting was cancelled.
2:15	potato chips	angry	I can't believe I am eating so much.
6:00	grilled shrimp, salad, asparagus, strawberries	happy	I chose a healthy dinner!
9:00	ice cream, cookies	lonely	No one called me tonight.
10:00	popcorn	lonely	Feeling very alone and empty.

To get you started, here's an easy-to-reference list of some of the uncomfortable feelings.

Afraid	Confused	Hurt
Angry	Embarrassed	Lonely
Ashamed	Guilty	Sad

Many other feelings exist, too, and are often connected to these major ones. Worried and anxious, for instance, are forms of fear; depressed and hopeless are types of sadness.

This gives you the general idea; now you can set up your own chart and begin to fill it in. If you are reading this in the afternoon or evening, it is perfectly okay for you to start now—it doesn't matter what time of day it is. If you are able, review your day to include earlier meals and snacks, thinking about what you ate and, if possible, what the feelings were as well as the precipitating events. If you can't identify the feeling or the pre-cipitating event, leave the space blank. Do your best, though, to fill in the chart as completely as possible. As you go through this book, it will become easier for you to recognize the stimulus (precipitating event) and to track your corresponding emotions.

I had been very uneducated about identifying feelings, and you might be in the same boat. Also, since emotional eaters use food to *not* feel, it might be very challenging to complete this chart. But don't worry about that right now. Fill in the chart to the best of your ability.

A side note: One of my pet peeves is hearing someone say, "I was bad—I ate such and such." What we eat has nothing to do with our moral character. If you do eat such and such, it just means you may have made a poor choice in food—it does not mean you are a bad person! When we judge ourselves as bad or naughty around our food, it some-times propels us to eat even more.

Day ③ Personal Journal

You are reading this book in order to stop emotional eating. Unless you allow yourself to feel your feelings and work through them, it will be very hard, if not impossible, to refrain from compulsive overeating. As you continue writing in your food-mood diary you will begin to recognize triggers. (In chapter 5, you will learn ways to dissipate the feelings and minimize the triggers.) Journaling is a way to encourage your feelings to come up, feelings that you've been running from. Use your notebook to create a personal journal for yourself and begin writing on a daily basis. With awareness can come change.

Many of my clients have told me that writing was one of the most important tools for getting them in touch with their feelings. Sometimes our conscious minds say one thing, but when we begin writing, we might be blown away at what comes forth. Journals are private, for your eyes only, and they allow you to express your emotions honestly.

Through writing, you can begin to explore some of the slippery feelings that are hard to define; you can clarify your feelings for yourself; you can have an emotional release. You will discover firsthand that when you discharge the feeling, the food craving disappears. Yes, that's right. When a feeling is bottled up, it can lead to food cravings or the need to fill up by compulsive overeating or bingeing. Once the emotion is released—by writing about it—the need for food subsides. It is quite amazing to experience this.

Journaling is also a great stress-management technique. You can write whatever you want and, as they say, let it all hang out. The journal is just for you; make sure you keep it in a safe place. Research has shown there are health benefits to journaling—it improves cognitive functioning, strengthens the immune system, lessens stress, helps clarify thoughts and feelings, and opens the way to understanding oneself better.

For many years, I kept a journal with my private thoughts and feelings. Many times I started a page with "I don't know what to write about today." But within a few minutes, my pen was gliding along the page, leaving a trail of words in its wake. When I allowed myself to feel whatever was bubbling up within me, I allowed the words to spill out on the page. I didn't care about spelling or punctuation, I just let my hand keep writing and writing until I felt spent. Spent, but happier. Writing was very therapeutic for me.

When I began journaling, I was afraid of examining my feelings. I had just started psychotherapy with the unspoken intention of figuring out why I was compelled to eat so much, and I was seeing my therapist twice a week. But my emotions had been pushed down for so long that I felt like Pandora's box—I was concerned that if I accessed those long-suppressed feelings, I'd never be able to close them off again. I feared touching into that dark pit of emotions would open me up too much and then our session would be over and I'd be left alone with my raw feelings. So instead of facing my feelings for the first time on someone else's schedule and with an audience, I went home after each therapy appointment and wrote in my journal. I wrote . . . I cried . . . I wrote some more . . . I cried some more. Each week I took my journal with me to my therapy session and read my tear-stained entries. Although I never allowed myself to cry during a session, the therapist and I talked about my feelings, and I received valuable counseling about what I had written.

Now as a psychotherapist myself, I have the opportunity to read and discuss clients' journals with them. Here is an excerpt from Lisa's journal. I shortened her actual entry (often the insights come after a page or two has been written):

> I am feeling so alone. No one called me yesterday and I didn't go out of the house. What's wrong with me? I am a mess. I am alone. I am me. I don't like me. No wonder no one comes to see me. Me. Me. Me. Me. Who am I? Who is me?
>
> I could just wither away and die and no one would notice. Well, I guess I won't wither away cuz I keep eating and eating. Why am I eating so much lately? I want to feel full. My life feels empty and food gives me fullness and satisfaction. But not really. It doesn't last. I eat and eat and eat. I like feeling stuffed. I hate feeling stuffed. I like feeling full. I hate it when my stomach hurts but I deserve to be in pain.
>
> I see it, maybe. I feel alone, I feel lonesome, I feel empty. No one calls. I am shut in. I open the cupboards and they are filled with my friends—they make me happy. I like crunching chips but then

my mouth feels scratchy and sore. . . . My mouth hurts, under my tongue. Why did I eat so many chips? They started tasting like oil but I didn't stop until the bag was empty. Then my mouth hurt and my lips were sore from the salt.

I ate so much yesterday that I was on the verge of feeling sick. How could I think of food as my friend? I felt so nauseous after all that I ate, but I couldn't stop. I went into some kind of trance I think. I don't even remember getting the chips out of the cupboard and then I was standing with an empty bag wiping salt off my lips.

What is wrong with me? Why do I keep eating and eating? Why am I so alone? Maybe I should join a church or a photo class or a meet-up group. It feels like too much work. I can stay home with my food or I can make myself go out and meet people. The food is so much easier. Let's see, what shall I choose—food or friends??? What would it take for me to go out and meet people? Why don't my friends call me more? Why am I always alone? That's not true, I am not always alone. I was alone yesterday. Last week I met Joan for dinner one night and had lunch with Sally. Last week Mo and I went to the show. Maybe I do see people. I didn't yesterday. Why didn't I call anyone?

Okay, I will do it. I will call Jean or Greta or Sue today and make a date to see them. I was having a pity party yesterday and turned to my old friends—chips and cookies. I felt like I was a little kid with no friends. I have friends. I forgot. *I have friends.* Maybe I don't see them or hear from them every day. Sometimes I like being alone and sometimes it makes me lonely. I have friends and we get along. Food is sometimes the only friend I know. I need to remember I have friends who aren't in the cupboard or refrigerator.

Lisa and I had been working together for several weeks at the point she wrote that entry, and she wrote in her journal almost every day. Although sometimes she continued to overeat and use food to fill her emptiness, Lisa was gaining insight into her emotional needs and why she was turning to food. When she first came to see me, her binges were at least once a day. Once she started journaling, she reported that the binges were much less frequent, sometimes not even once a week. As we looked at her writing together, she began to understand what was going on in herself before she binged.

Assignment

It is important to express somewhere what you are feeling so you don't end up eating because of it. Journaling is one of the best personal-growth practices for emotional clarity, so get in the habit of writing in your journal daily, for at least ten minutes. Opening up in this way can be a deep, cathartic experience. You will discover the magic of journaling as you write what's going on for you, on the inside, honestly.

If you don't know where to start, you could begin with "What is bothering me today?" or "Why do I eat so much?" or "What makes me happy?" or "I am really angry about _____." And, if all else fails, just write, "I don't know what to write" over and over again. The important thing is to keep writing.

Your entries will probably be a lot different than Lisa's—everyone is unique, and every journal entry is different. There is no need for any specific structure—just begin using the tool of writing and see what comes out. Write quickly, without censoring yourself; don't worry about spelling and punctuation. Great writing is not required, only a desire to uncover hidden feelings and get to the core of your being.

Begin to trigger old memories using photographs, old address books, or other memory-joggers. Getting honest is the first step in reducing the bingeing as you move toward the goal of self-acceptance. We all eat because we are hungry. Now you are beginning to identify the hunger. It is often not physical, but an emotional or spiritual hunger.

You are not alone. You are not the only person who has felt this way or used food in this way. It is important to have a support system, which we'll talk about next.

Chapter 3

Finding Support

> No one can whistle a symphony.
> It takes a whole orchestra to play it.
> —H. E. LUCCOCK, METHODIST EPISCOPAL CHURCH BISHOP

YOU ARE NOW WRITING IN your food-mood diary every day, as well as journaling your feelings. As you continue with these activities, chances are really good that you will begin to have insights and aha moments. But since these are both solitary endeavors, it is time to also create a support system to ensure you get encouragement and strength from others. Moreover, you need to become your own advocate, your own cheerleader, as you learn to take better care of yourself. This chapter touches on both these aspects—creating an outside support system as well as learning to support and nurture yourself. In addition, Day 6 deals with seeking professional help, if needed.

Day ④ Creating a Support System

Often we are our own worst enemies. I vividly remember a poignant Ziggy cartoon illustrating the truth of this statement. In the first frame we see Ziggy, with head bowed, and the caption "God grant me one request—destroy my worst enemy." The next frame is a large lightning bolt and the word ZAP! The third frame displays a pile of ashes with smoke rising and the words "Let me rephrase that!"

Yes, we can each be our own worst enemy. As you do the inner work necessary to curb emotional eating, it is crucial to encircle yourself with supportive people. While you will have the outlet of writing in your journal, it is also important to have someone to confide in. Then, if you fall into old patterns with food, you'll have someone to talk to about it. A typical response from your Inner Critic is blaming and shaming, which can lead to more self-loathing and more binge eating. A nonjudgmental friend, however, might acknowledge those feelings and then help you move past them with a fresh perspective and positive actions.

Surround yourself with friends or family members who care about you and want what's best for you. Having a support system is like having a safety net below you at all times. It gives you the courage to take the next step forward, and then the next, as you embark on this journey of self-discovery and transformation.

Likewise, it is essential that you avoid people who might sabotage your efforts—those who discourage you from changing or who actively bring you unhealthy food as treats. Identify individuals who are critical, cause you to feel bad about yourself, or drain your energy—and stay away from them. Choose instead to hang out with those who applaud your efforts, who celebrate you for being you, and who are trustworthy with your feelings.

When I was at my lowest emotionally, I was fortunate to find Twelve-Step meetings. The openness and self-honesty I heard in the rooms were both foreign and frightening to me. Even so, I returned week after week because I saw, for the first time, people who had lost weight and were keeping it off. Over two hundred different self-help groups, with a combined worldwide membership of millions, now employ Twelve-Step principles for recovery. This book's Resources section offers more information about some of the food-related recovery groups.

When I stopped eating compulsively, I began to experience a hodgepodge of feelings. The Twelve-Step meetings provided a support system where I began to let others in, allowing them to see the real me by sharing my innermost thoughts, along with the fragile, newfound feelings that accompanied them. Later, I sponsored other people, assisting them in ending their own obsession with food.

It took me a while to understand the program, and applying the steps became my first experience with personal-growth work. The original Twelve Steps, as set by Alcoholics Anonymous, state:

Step 1: We admitted we were powerless over alcohol—that our lives had become unmanageable [In food-related programs, *alcohol* is replaced with *food*, etc.]

Step 2: Came to believe that a Power greater than ourselves could restore us to sanity

Step 3: Made a decision to turn our will and our lives over to the care of God *as we understood Him* [Many groups have changed *Him* to *God* to make it gender neutral. To make the statements originally including *God* more religiously neutral, the word can be changed to *a Higher Power*, or something similar. The Twelve-Step groups listed in the Resources are not religious but are spiritual and open to people of all religions, and of no religions, including atheists and agnostics.]

Step 4: Made a searching and fearless moral inventory of ourselves

Step 5: Admitted to God, to ourselves, and to another human being the exact nature of our wrongs

Step 6: Were entirely ready to have God remove all these defects of character

Step 7: Humbly asked Him to remove our shortcomings

Step 8: Made a list of all persons we had harmed, and became willing to make amends to them all

Step 9: Made direct amends to such people wherever possible, except when to do so would injure them or others

Step 10: Continued to take personal inventory and when we were wrong promptly admitted it

Step 11: Sought through prayer and meditation to improve our conscious contact with God, *as we understood Him,* praying only for knowledge of His will for us and the power to carry that out

Step 12: Having had a spiritual awakening as the result of these steps, we tried to carry this message to others, and to practice these principles in all our affairs

My journey to health, my life without compulsive overeating, began with Twelve-Step Recovery, which combines spiritual, emotional, mental, and physical recovery. If you are struggling with food, I urge you to check out a few of the meetings.

Some people balk because of the mention of God in the steps—but please don't let that deter you. People of all religions, as wells as agnostics and atheists, have benefitted from these fellowships. Overeaters Anonymous (OA) was the first, and many others have sprung up. Below is a list of some of them. For descriptions, go to the Resources section at the end of the book.

Anorexics and Bulimics Anonymous (ABA)
www.aba12steps.org

Compulsive Eaters Anonymous-HOW (CEA-HOW)
www.ceahow.org

Eating Addictions Anonymous (EAA)
www.eatingaddictionsanonymous.org

Eating Disorders Anonymous (EDA)
www.eatingdisordersanonymous.org

Food Addicts Anonymous (FAA)
www.foodaddictsanonymous.org

Food Addicts in Recovery Anonymous (FA)
www.foodaddicts.org

GreySheeters Anonymous (GSA)
www.greysheet.org

Overeaters Anonymous (OA)
www.oa.org

Since the Twelve-Step approach does not appeal to everyone, you might choose to find your support elsewhere, and that's fine. Search online or ask trusted friends and healthcare professionals for self-help groups near you and for other resources. Online chat rooms and forums can be particularly helpful because they are always "open." Someone is always listening and trying to help. Here are a few online sources to get you started:

www.MentorConnect-ed.org is designed to replace eating disorders with relationships. It is the first global online mentoring community which provides one-on-one matches for individuals seeking recovery.

www.EatingDisorderRecovery.com, an extensive website containing articles that support, inform, and encourage recovery, was created by Joanna Poppink, psychotherapist and author of *Healing Your Hungry Heart.*

www.BEDAonline.org provides individuals who suffer from binge eating disorder with resources to begin a safe journey toward a healthy recovery.

www.HealthyGirl.org is an online support site for girls and young women who binge or emotionally overeat.

www.Something-Fishy.org is dedicated to raising awareness and providing support for people with eating disorders and has a directory of treatment providers and support groups.

www.NationalEatingDisorders.org offers support groups, advice, and referrals.

Another option is to join a group that offers general support for expressing yourself honestly and receiving empathy. The Center for Nonviolent Communication (CNVC) provides such groups. Nonviolent communication (NVC), which can also be understood as compassionate communication, was originally developed in the 1960s by Dr. Marshall Rosenberg, an American psychologist. It is a process of communication based on transforming our judgments into feelings and needs. During NVC classes and seminars, students discover how to give compassionate responses to themselves and others based on the feelings and needs beneath the words.

For those of us who have berated ourselves for years, NVC is an excellent way to learn to be more empathetic. When I studied NVC, I found the process of self-empathy very challenging at first. I couldn't forgive myself for having what I saw as gargantuan warts. It took a lot of practice for me to become gentle and forgiving of myself, but I eventually noticed that calling myself stupid had (mostly) stopped. Now, when I goof up, I call myself silly. Unlike the word *stupid,* the word *silly* is light and almost humorous, and hearing it doesn't feel like I've been punched in the gut. Rather than seeing my human foibles as so darn serious, *silly* allows me to lighten up and even laugh at myself from time to time.

Finding supportive people or a support group meets our very important need to belong. Lynne McTaggart discusses this crucial need in her book *The Bond*:

> The need to move beyond the boundaries of ourselves as individuals and to bond with a group is so primordial and necessary to human beings that it remains the key determinant of whether we remain healthy or get ill, even whether we live or die. It is more vital to us than any diet or exercise program. The Bond we make with a group is the most fundamental need we have because it generates our most authentic state of being.

Assignment

Start investigating various Twelve-Step groups. Find meetings in your area, and make a commitment to yourself to attend at least one meeting within the next week. The feeling of belonging might not happen immediately—I often heard others say they felt as if they were home at their first meeting, but I had to attend many, many meetings before I began to feel connected to the group—but it's worth your while to try.

If you have already been exposed to Twelve-Step Recovery and decided it is not right for you, then be sure to check out other possible self-help or support groups. In addition, begin identifying people with whom you can allow yourself to be vulnerable, sharing the real you. Find a buddy with whom you check in every day. Since creating a strong support system takes time, it is wise to begin the process today.

Day ⑤ Self-Care

In addition to creating a support system of caring people around you, it is time to stop being your own worst enemy and begin to become your own best friend. Let's start with ways you can take better care of yourself. As a psychotherapist, I see time and time again the adverse effects of my clients' lack of self-care. In general, women have been conditioned to be the givers, but men aren't very good at making themselves a priority, either.

Do you put everyone else's needs before your own? What do you do to take care of yourself? Are you finding time to play? To laugh? To relax? To nurture yourself? The chances are pretty good that you are not—at least not yet. But with the help of some simple tools, that can—and will—change.

In days long ago, I was always more interested in assisting others than in taking care of myself. I didn't ever want to appear selfish, so I continued to give and give of myself until eventually the well ran dry. While being selfish can mean being stingy, exercising self-care is filling yourself up *before,* not *instead of,* giving to others. I was thrilled to discover that when I spent time caring for myself first, I had far more energy for others.

Every time we're on an airplane, we hear some version of the following: "In case of a sudden drop in pressure, the oxygen masks will appear. Put your own mask on first and then assist others." What is true for literal oxygen masks in singular emergencies is also true for metaphorical ones in daily life. We can't really support others unless we are taking care of ourselves. I remind my clients (and sometimes myself) over and over again: Put on your own oxygen mask first, and then you will have something to give.

In addition, how many of us lead our lives doing what we think we *should* do or what we think we *have to* do? During my childhood and young adulthood, I did whatever I thought I was supposed to do. I dreamed about finding a giant book of rules so I could be certain to live my life according to the *shoulds* and not make *any* mistakes! The external voices of my parents and teachers told me what I should do, such as "You should go to bed now" or "You should be nice all the time," and what I should not do, like "You should not show anger" or "You should not be fat." I internalized these voices, and soon my own inner voice was barking commands at me: *You should go to sleep. You should smile more. You should not eat those cookies. You should be ashamed of yourself. You should lose weight.* My inner world, the voices in my head, became a constant chatter of *shoulds* and *should nots*—about everything!

During my journey of recovery, I found authors and lecturers who helped me change my self-talk, with suggestions such as "You shouldn't *should* on yourself." The motivational author Louise Hay suggests we change our *shoulds* to *coulds*. When I catch myself saying *I should*, I quickly correct it to *I could* and am amazed at how quickly my disposition improves. Try it—you'll see what I mean. *I could go to sleep. I could smile more. I could be nice all the time.* It really feels different.

This is also true for the words *have to*. I used to say to myself, *I have to make dinner. I have to pick up the kids from school. I have to exercise. I have to go on a diet.* The part of me that is a rebel didn't want to be told what I have to do—so sometimes I would simply not do it. Other times I would do it with the attitude of a victim—*Oh, poor me, I have to pick up the kids from school.* Try changing each *have to* to *choose to.* What a difference this makes—when we change the words, we change the energy. *I choose to make dinner. I choose to pick up the kids from school. I choose to exercise.* The word *choose* dissipates that poor-me voice and the feeling of being a victim and leads instead to feelings of self-empowerment. And the good news is, the stronger we feel, the weaker the compulsion to overeat.

Assignment

Since it is important to take better care of yourself, what activities are you willing to add (on a daily basis) to nurture yourself? Here are some ideas:

- Indulge in a bath with candles or bath salts
- Laugh
- Pour yourself a cup of tea and relax for five minutes
- Do nothing for five minutes without the cup of tea
- Go outside and tune in to the wonders of nature
- Read a book just for pleasure
- Take a leisurely walk
- Do some deep breathing
- Do five minutes of stretching or yoga
- Pamper yourself (Massage? Pedicure?)
- Spend time enjoying your favorite hobby
- Engage in a social activity you enjoy
- Hang out with a friend
- Watch a funny movie
- Watch a sitcom on TV
- Listen to music
- Sing
- Dance
- Play with your pet
- Take a nap
- Peruse photos that bring back wonderful memories
- Stargaze
- Buy yourself some flowers

- Watch some fun YouTube videos
- Pick a flower and examine the intricacies of the petals
- Hum or whistle a favorite tune

Each day you can pick a different activity. It's your choice. Be creative—you are not limited to this list. Do whatever feels nurturing to you, and make it a habit to give yourself at least five minutes a day.

◆

Write down at least ten things you think you have to do or should do. Your list might look like this:

1. I have to clean the house.
2. I have to prepare meals.
3. I have to pay bills.
4. I should lose weight.
5. I should call my parents.
6. I should take a walk, etc.

Read it aloud. Then change each *have to* to *choose to*, each *should* to *could*.

Original List	Revised List
I have to clean the house.	I choose to clean the house.
I have to prepare meals.	I choose to prepare meals.
I have to pay bills.	I choose to pay bills.
I should lose weight.	I could lose weight.
I should call my parents.	I could call my parents.
I should take a walk.	I could take a walk.

Read the revised list out loud. It carries a different energy than the first list and should (oops, did I use that word?!) feel very freeing.

Your ongoing assignment is to become more conscious of the words you use, so when you hear yourself say (perhaps in a whiny tone) "I have to make dinner," you will catch yourself immediately and change it to "I choose to make dinner." And in so doing, you will find yourself feeling far more content and empowered in your everyday life.

Day 6 Therapy

Many compulsive overeaters are able to stop the obsession simply by using the various tools discussed throughout this book. For others, it might be necessary to see a psychotherapist to explore and work on the feelings and issues that drive the repeated episodes of binge eating.

In my family, we didn't believe in psychotherapy—we didn't want to air our dirty laundry in public, and besides, we assumed we didn't have any dirty laundry to air! My entrance into the world of therapy became necessary because of my young daughter's reaction to having a baby brother. When I gave birth to my son, my three-year-old daughter began to act out her jealousy. In addition, as my son became mobile, she started to experience separation anxiety—I could not leave her at preschool until she felt safe and secure, with her tiny little hand firmly enclosed in the hand of her teacher. I asked our pediatrician for a recommendation, and although he was a very body-focused practitioner, he suggested I go to a psychotherapist. Since it involved my daughter's emotional well-being, I agreed to go at once. I didn't think I needed therapy, but I was willing to see someone because my child had pressing issues.

At the first appointment, Jean Kushleika (the recommended social worker) informed me that instead of seeing my daughter directly, she preferred to work with me—the parent—first, and then have me work with my daughter. I smiled and said, "Of course I'll come in and see you." Inside, though, I was screaming. I knew my number was up—someone would soon see what a terrible fraud I was.

I began seeing the social worker every week. She gave me permission to have feelings and provided a safe place to share them; she taught me to allow my children to show their feelings, too. Wow, what a concept—to have and express feelings! I took notes during our sessions. At home I would ask my daughter to sit next to me on the couch, and I'd read my notes to her: "Mommy thinks you're angry," or whatever emotion the therapist had suggested, given the circumstances.

One day I reported to Mrs. Kushleika that my daughter was displaying inappropriate anger with her little brother. I was astounded at the therapist's response: "Your daughter will not learn to deal with her anger until you deal with yours."

What?! Me, angry? I'm not angry! I screamed inside my head. I had resolved long ago to never be angry. It was a conscious decision. I could be nice, or I could be angry, and I chose to be nice. So what in the world was she talking about?

Thus began my journey into understanding myself—into identifying the suppressed feelings and the masks I wore. I was terrified—someone was beginning to understand me. I was elated—someone was beginning to understand me.

Psychotherapy was real work for me as I kept digging deeper and deeper into aspects of myself I had buried for years. Slowly I became conscious of the individual I was inside. I didn't want to know at first—I was sure I was a bad person, a monster in some ways. I had not yet recognized there were any positives about me, and the negatives were unmistakable from my point of view. It took a lot of courage for me to acknowledge all those facets of myself that I had successfully avoided for so long.

Although terrified at the outset to reveal myself in therapy, it turned out to be one of the best decisions I ever made. Boy, was it intense work—and life changing! I went twice a week for a while, opening up bit by bit. I felt like an explorer discovering what made me tick. As I continued therapy, the critical voice playing in my head became less ferocious and less frequent. I often thought I needed to be faultless, but my therapist reiterated again and again that I just needed to be "good enough." After several years in therapy, I emerged feeling whole and complete, with a lot more self-understanding and self-acceptance than I had ever had before.

Psychotherapy is a wonderful adjunct to any personal-growth path. As compulsive overeaters, we use food to ease emotional discomfort and fill up the emptiness within. Take away our drug of choice, give up the binges, and what is often left is a life filled with pain. Therapy is a necessary

Stop Eating Your Heart Out

tool in these instances. We would not be using and misusing food, booze, or whatever our drug of choice might be if we could face life on life's terms without our crutches.

Assignment

Spend some time asking yourself if you need additional help to deal with your issues, and if so, begin to explore therapy options. For those with a history of rape or sexual abuse, it is not unusual to turn to food, and it is important to get outside help. If you are severely depressed, it is a good idea to seek a therapist. Also, many people find they need the help of residential, or inpatient, treatment where they can learn to change their relationship with food as they work through the underlying issues.

As you continue to explore and use the tools presented here, be open to the possibility that additional therapy might be helpful for you. Going to a therapist is not a sign of failure; it is an indication that you are willing to tackle the hard stuff so you can finally break free of the food obsession. In selecting a mental health provider, ask your friends and health-care professionals for a referral. It is okay to interview several therapists before selecting the one you want to work with. It needs to be someone you feel comfortable with, someone with whom you feel safe enough to reveal the real you.

With six days' worth of tools, you are now:

1. Aware of your eating history
2. Logging your food and feelings

3. Writing in your journal every day

4. Starting to develop a support system for yourself

5. Nurturing yourself, at least a few minutes every day

6. Understanding the benefits and importance of psychotherapy

The next chapter discusses support in another realm—increasing your spiritual connection, practicing meditation, and discovering the usefulness of creative visualization.

Chapter 4

Spirituality and Spiritual Growth

Just as a candle cannot burn without fire, men cannot live without a spiritual life.

—BUDDHA

AT SOME POINT EARLY IN my work with emotional eaters, I often ask them about their spiritual or religious beliefs. "What does spirituality have to do with my compulsive overeating?" they often ask. I explain that for many of us, emotional eating is due to a spiritual hunger, a hunger for a deeper meaning to life—and we're attempting to fill that void with food. In fact, current research shows that spiritual approaches (such as meditation and prayer) in the treatment of eating disorders are at least as effective (and sometimes more effective) than secular ones. Additionally, those in Twelve-Step Recovery learn that although the pressure to overeat might be emotional, the solution is spiritual. It is fitting, therefore, that as you pursue freedom from emotional eating, you at least explore your spirituality and contemplate what being spiritual means to you.

What does *spiritual* even mean? *Merriam-Webster* *.com* defines *spiritual* as:

of, relating to, consisting of, or affecting the spirit <*spiritual* needs>

of or relating to sacred matters <*spiritual* songs>; ecclesiastical rather than lay or temporal <*spiritual* authority>

concerned with religious values

related or joined in spirit <our *spiritual* home> <his *spiritual* heir>

of or relating to supernatural beings or phenomena: of, relating to, or involving spiritualism

Before you atheists and agnostics run, I ask you to consider that spirituality and religion are not one and the same. What I'm talking about is spirituality, not necessarily religiosity. The way I see it, organized religion often separates people (look at all the wars fought in the name of religion, for heaven's sake), whereas spirituality often unifies people by overlooking differences and showcasing commonalities.

Since the term *spirituality* is nebulous—it's the kind of thing we "get" but that's hard to put into words—let's take a look at what others have said about it. Rachel Naomi Remen, one of the first doctors to recognize the role of the spirit in health and wellness, declared:

[T]he spiritual is inclusive. It is the deepest sense of belonging and participation. We all participate in the spiritual at all times, whether we know it or not.

There's no place to go to be separated from the spiritual, so perhaps one might say that the spiritual is that realm of human experience which religion attempts to connect us to through dogma and practice. Sometimes it succeeds and sometimes it fails. Religion is a bridge to the spiritual—but the spiritual lies beyond religion. Unfortunately, in seeking the spiritual we may become attached to the bridge rather than crossing over it.

The most important thing in defining spirit is the recognition that the spirit is an essential need of human nature. There is something in all of us that seeks the spiritual. This yearning varies in strength from person to person but it is always there in everyone.

John-Roger, an international lecturer guiding people to find the spirit within, believes

You do not have to try to become spiritual. You don't have to try to be what you already are. The process of trying is like using a double negative; it's redundant. In a sense, trying to be spiritual is like a female trying to be female. She already is; it's not necessary to try. She might "try" to match her expression with some outer criteria or someone's opinion, but that she is a female is a fact. Men and women are spiritual beings. They do not have to try to become that. To express that spirituality consciously in day-to-day activities may be a little bit different. They may have to work to express that quality more directly.

(The Way Out Book, 28–29)

Father Leo Booth, a Unity minister, speaker, and author, and well-known in the recovery community, explained,

We associate spirit with positive and creative energy. This energy gives us the power to live, work, and create. Spiritual people are positive and creative human beings. They know, deep inside themselves, that they have the power to create the difference in their lives. They have looked within and found what can be called their yes to life, and this yes shines forth in their attitudes and actions.

(When God Becomes a Drug, 56)

As we discuss spirituality throughout this book, we will see it directly linked to personal growth. Spirituality can connect us deeply to our core or spirit, take us to the depths of our inner being, and include our search for life's meaning and purpose. I have observed that as one's spirituality gets stronger, the food obsession becomes weaker.

With that said, let's find ways to increase your spirituality, if you so choose!

Day ⑦ Higher Power

In chapter 3, we discussed the importance of having a support system, and now we broaden it to include spiritual support. Perhaps you already have a great relationship with a Higher Power. But maybe you don't. In this section I share my challenges with the notion of God and offer ways for you to develop and strengthen a relationship for yourself with the Higher Power of your choice.

It took me many years to recognize that spirituality is all-inclusive and can bring people of different faiths together. As a third grader, I was required to attend vesper services. Although these are nondenominational, I felt as if I was being forced to go to church, and I wrote in my diary: "Today we went to vesper services, but I didn't sing or pray because it is against my religion."

Much later, when I started attending Twelve-Step meetings, which are almost always held in churches, I joked that the "church people" were out to convert me. During the meetings, every time they said the *G* word—*God*— I snickered or turned to my friend and rolled my eyes. I hated hearing the *G* word. Behind the jokes, I actually did fear that people were trying to convert me. I was so turned off I almost didn't go back to another meeting.

For years I proclaimed I was agnostic—I didn't know if God existed or not. At least that is what I told myself. In reality, I wanted to be agnostic because I was afraid of

God—all I knew was a punishing God, one who "knows if you've been bad or good, so be good for goodness' sake."

I had spent years and years convincing others of my goodness, and I excelled in the role of Miss Goody Two-Shoes: I acted righteous, followed the rules, and did what I was told (except for sneak eating and sneak smoking). But my insides didn't match my outsides. I would do and say everything right, but I knew, and therefore God knew, about all the things I did that weren't good—what I refer to as my "little bads." For example, I might compliment an older relative by saying "That's a beautiful hat," but mocking words often reverberated inside my head, and I could actually be thinking "What a ridiculous-looking hat."

Additionally, I always acted loving toward my siblings, especially my brother (six years younger than I). But there were a few times when I did unloving things to him. For instance, many years before the movie *A Christmas Story* came out, I suggested he put his lip on the ice-cube tray. When it stuck and ripped off some skin, I played the innocent: "Oh, you poor thing. I didn't know that would happen." Another time, when I was nine and he was three, the family went swimming at an outdoor pool. I saw a bee land on my towel. In a sugary-sweet voice, I asked my brother to bring me my towel. My loving, devoted little brother picked up the towel, and the bee stung him. I acted blameless and with all the sincerity I could muster offered, "Oh, you poor thing, I didn't know there was a bee on the towel."

As I grew into adulthood, I continued the charade, endeavoring to always look good and say the right thing. Inside, though, I continually criticized and judged others and myself. Although I always acted nice, no one knew about the horde of insults traipsing through my mind. But I knew. And I feared God did, too. I considered myself a phony, and God knew about the deception. In fact, the God I was so afraid to believe in was watching me and keeping track—noting such things as Insincere Compliment Number 983.

Of course I didn't want to believe in God. My God was a punishing God who knew me as deceitful, dishonest, and a hypocrite. As the television character Maude used to say, "He'll get you for that!" I could, at any time, receive some big-time punishment; I was terrified of God's wrath and the horrible consequences that awaited me for being such a fake.

As a young married woman, I lived a tormented life: I had two healthy children (first a girl, then a boy—just what I wanted); I had a successful husband, a lovely home, and no financial worries. But some day I knew I would receive the punishment I deserved from the God I believed in. My greatest moments of inner agony occurred after giving birth to my healthy second child—*now it might be payback time.* And what better way to get back at a mom than through her children. Each day, I awoke fraught with fear wondering, *Is today the day God will strike one of my children with an incurable disease?* What angst. What pain.

After months of this living hell, I attended a Twelve-Step weekend and heard the keynote speaker say, "God loves me no matter what!" Those six words opened a new door for me. Well, maybe it was a window, just a crack, but it was an opening to begin to revise my perception of God.

Unconditional love? What a concept! I listened intently to the speaker, who was totally convinced that he didn't have to do anything to be loved—he just was. I absorbed his words and, little by little, came to slowly change my view of God from one of punishment and retribution to one of unconditional love.

Here is a letter I wrote a long, long time ago, when I was first becoming aware of my spirituality:

Dear Higher Power,

Thank you for always being with me. Sometimes, though, I can't feel you at all and sometimes I don't like my life that you gave me. I know I should feel grateful but I am hurting inside. I feel very alone. I want someone to hold my hand and walk with me.

Someone on the earth plane—you are not on the physical plane and it isn't enough for me. When I am feeling sad, I wish there was someone who would wipe my tears, pat me on the back, tell me that I am doing a good job, and just love me for being me. I really want that and I want that now. You are out there, I know, but I want more than the God in the sky kind of love. I need love and companionship and I need it now.

I am tired of being fat. I am still eating too much. Too much and too fast. I feel so empty inside. Can I believe that you will fill the emptiness? How is that possible? Food no longer works for me but it is the only thing I know. I want to believe in you and that you are taking care of me but I have such an ache inside and I don't let anyone know about it. Please help me, Higher Power. Please take away my pain and suffering. I believe you can do it. Will you? Please, please, please!

As I wrote the letter I felt sad and desperate, on the edge of hopelessness. Somehow, though, putting the words to paper and appealing to a Higher Power helped release some of my feelings. After I finished the letter, I just sat and breathed deeply for a few moments. A sense of peace came over me.

Opening to a loving Higher Power, whom I now choose to call God (this took me a very long while to get used to), has allowed me to feel permeated with God's love. I no longer believe in a punishing God—my Higher Power loves me no matter what. I am profoundly grateful I had a spiritual awakening. Instead of the fear I once felt, now I only feel love.

There are a lot of people who are challenged with the word *God* and the connotations it carries. Some folks were raised in strict religious homes and resist the many rules and demands once made of them. Others grew up in homes devoid of any religion and were taught that there is no such thing as God. Many people have no idea that spirituality can exist apart from organized religion, and since they have turned away from religion, they cannot imagine how they can pursue spirituality.

As a counselor working with people in recovery, I find spirituality to be an important part of the work we do together. Some clients have had challenges with this. Julia, for instance, was a product of Catholic schools and had her knuckles whacked with a ruler way too often. Upon graduation, she got as far away from the church as she could. At our first session, Julia stated that she wanted to work on weight issues and emphatically declared that she was not religious and wanted nothing to do with God.

Probing a bit, I asked Julia if there was anything she could believe in that was bigger than herself that she could make her Higher Power. I suggested that sometimes people feel a connection to nature. The following week Julia reported that she had been spending some time outdoors—meandering through a park—and felt very peaceful there. She agreed that she could use nature as her Higher Power. As Julia worked on her emotional eating issues, she very successfully leaned on and felt supported by this Higher Power.

Perhaps you, too, have a negative reaction to the word *God*. Or maybe you have a strong connection to God, or Jesus, or Buddha, or Jehovah, or Allah. Since there are so many beliefs, I use words like *Universe, Spirit, Source, Loving Presence, the Divine,* or *Creator* to refer to whomever or whatever we believe in. Sometimes I also use the term *Higher Self* to denote that part of yourself that is spiritual and connected to all that is.

For those of us who are compulsive overeaters, Food has become our God, our Higher Power. It is larger than us, more powerful than us, and it can transform us. It is time to fire that Higher Power and begin to allow Food to just be food and not your god. It is imperative that your Higher Power be something outside yourself, bigger than you, which symbolizes or expresses unconditional love.

As emotional eaters, we tend to isolate and feel alone. Developing and strengthening our connection to Spirit can allow us to feel supported even during those alone times. Many of us discover that as we deepen our spiritual connection, the comfort we used to receive from food is replaced by the comfort we receive from our Higher Power.

Assignment

For those who are challenged to find a Higher Power, try choosing something such as nature to be your Higher Power. Be in nature. If possible, take a walk and use as many senses as you can. Explore the landscape. Stop and look at a blade of grass or the opening of a flower. Examine it and tune in with your senses: Notice colors, shapes, sizes, smells, and textures. Do you feel a sense of peace when you're in nature? You might want to use nature as (part of) your Higher Power.

◆

Carve out some quiet time in a quiet place and write a letter to your Higher Power/God/Source/Universe. Your Higher Power needs to be a Loving Presence. Again, if it is a punishing deity, please oust that one and get a new one that is all-loving. Open your heart and express your wants, your hopes, your needs, and your frustrations. After completing the letter, allow yourself to just sit and breathe for a few minutes.

Day ⑧ Prayer and Meditation

It's been said that prayer is us talking to Spirit, and meditation is our being still and listening. Prayer can be an act of reading words from sacred texts or forming words from your own heart. As your personal communication with the Divine, prayer is about obtaining, maintaining, and fostering a relationship with that Higher Power. My clients have been thrilled to find that the more time they put into prayer and meditation, the less pull there has been to compulsively eat. For many, a quick prayer when the food is beckoning ("Please, God, keep me out of the kitchen") has prevented a binge from happening.

Prayer

Prayers are often taught in childhood and have a place in many homes of the very religious as well as the not-so-religious. For instance, every night I was taught to say this classic children's prayer:

> Now I lay me down to sleep,
> I pray the Lord my soul to keep.
> And if I die before I wake,
> I pray the Lord my soul to take.

I then learned to add "God bless Mommy and Daddy, my brother and sister, my grandmothers, my cousins, my aunts and uncles," mentioning specific names. I didn't know what the prayer meant, but I faithfully recited it every night because it was expected of me.

Many folks brought up in Christian homes know by heart the Lord's Prayer:

Our Father, who art in heaven, hallowed be thy
name.
Thy kingdom come, thy will be done, on earth as
it is in heaven.
Give us this day our daily bread.
And forgive us our trespasses, as we forgive those
who trespass against us.
And lead us not into temptation, but deliver us
from evil.
For thine is the kingdom, the power, and the glory,
forever and ever.
Amen.

I am very familiar with the Lord's Prayer because it is frequently recited at Twelve-Step meetings, but the predominant prayer that flows through my head comes from the Jewish tradition—the Shema:

Šěma' Yisrā'el Ădōnāy Ēlōhênû Ădōnāy eḥād.

That is, of course, the transliteration. The English translation is:

Hear, O Israel, the Lord is our God, the Lord is One.

Prayers abound in Twelve-Step Recovery rooms, and each meeting usually includes the Serenity Prayer, written by Reinhold Niebuhr:

God, grant me the serenity
To accept the things I cannot change;
Courage to change the things I can;
And wisdom to know the difference.

Two more prayers became extremely important to me as I worked the Twelve Steps. The Third Step Prayer is one that I still recite a lot because it takes me outside myself, trusting in a loving, all-knowing Higher Power to take over.

God, I offer myself to Thee—to build with me and to do with me as Thou wilt. Relieve me of the bondage of self, that I may better do Thy will. Take away my difficulties, that victory over them may bear witness to those I would help of Thy Power, Thy Love, and Thy Way of life. May I do Thy will always!

I start most days with this prayer, and I repeat these words over and over again throughout the day—when I want to connect to Spirit, before seeing clients, as I prepare to teach, on my morning walk, or when I am driving the car.

When I discovered the Seventh Step Prayer, I was more than a little relieved to learn that I can offer my whole self to my Higher Power. Silly me, I thought I had to be flawless to be of use! I was flabbergasted to find out that even my faults were of value and the only character defects I needed to change were those that prevented me from being useful to my Higher Power and others.

My Creator, I am now willing that you should have all of me, good and bad. I pray that you now remove from me every single defect of character which stands in the way of my usefulness to you and my fellows. Grant me strength, as I go out from here to do your bidding. Amen.

Stop Eating Your Heart Out

In addition to written prayers, we often say our own personal, impromptu prayers:

- Prayers of petition (this is what I want or need)
- Prayers of thanksgiving and gratitude (thankfulness for all that I have been given)
- Prayers for others (I pray for a loved one's recovery)
- Prayers of repentance (I messed up and I am truly sorry)
- Conversational prayers (talking to or having a conversation with Spirit in my mind).

Meditation

If prayer is speaking to Spirit, meditation is being still enough to hear the voice of that Loving Presence. Meditation quiets the mind, relaxes the body, and helps us to focus on the present. Once the head chatter has stopped, you are open to experiencing guidance or inner wisdom and might intuitively get an answer to a question that has plagued you. I like Joan Borysenko's simple definition: "Meditation is any activity that keeps the attention pleasantly anchored in the present moment" (*Minding the Body, Mending the Mind,* 36). Although there are different types of meditation, most include the following:

> **Quiet.** When new to meditation, it is helpful to be in a location without distractions (phone, TV, others talking) where you will not be disturbed.

> **Comfort.** You do not need to be sitting like a yogi to experience meditation. It is often

recommended, however, that you keep your spine straight. If you tend to nod off, be seated rather than lying down.

Concentration. You can gaze at an object (maybe one in nature—a leaf, waves of the ocean, a tree in the distance—or perhaps something like the flame of a candle). You can repeat a mantra—a sound, a syllable, a word such as *Om*, or *Love*, or *One*. Focus on your breathing. When your mind wanders, gently bring it back to your focal point.

Observation. Rather than judging yourself, be in the role of detached observer. No judgments, no criticisms—just notice with impartiality.

Awareness of the breath. Many meditations begin by placing your attention on your breathing. As you do so, you become more and more relaxed. If this is new to you (or even if it's not), you can try out the following meditation.

Conscious Breathing Meditation

Sit with your spine straight and your feet flat on the floor. Wiggle around a little and then settle in. Allow your tongue to gently rest behind your top front teeth. Become aware of your breath. Focus on the inhale and the exhale. Feel the breath. Where do you feel it in your body? Are you aware of sounds as the breath goes in or goes out? Just be aware of the breath—don't change it. Just notice it.

As you are breathing, thoughts might pop into your head. Put these thoughts on clouds and let them float by, as you gently bring your attention back to your breath. Stay with the breath, shifting your awareness back to it when you drift into thought. Put your hands on your belly and feel it rise when you inhale. (Many people only breathe to the top of the lungs—it is important to bring your breath down low so that you feel your belly expand like a balloon on the inhale and deflate on the exhale. It can take a little practice to do this.)

Now breathe in through your nose, pause, and breathe out through your mouth. As you inhale, count. Pause. Exhale and count. Pause. This time, allow your exhalation to last two counts longer than your inhalation—for example, if you inhale to the count of four, exhale to the count of six:

1. Inhale (count) through your nose.
2. Pause.
3. Exhale (count + 2) through your mouth.
4. Pause.
5. Repeat. Repeat. Repeat.

Ignore thoughts and distractions, and continue to bring your awareness back to the breath. Clear your mind. Heighten your senses. Be still. Breathe.

Not all meditation involves stillness. Many people find repetitive activities, such as knitting, gardening, ironing, washing the dishes, or walking, very soothing and use them as meditative practices.

Walking Meditation

This is an active meditation process in which the very act of walking is the focus.

When you try this, pay attention to your body as you walk: the feeling of the ground beneath your feet, the bend of your knees as you take a step, the movement of your arms as they gently swing at your sides, the breath as it goes in and out, the movement of your belly. Continue to notice any body sensations. Is there tightness in your chest? Are your eyes squinting in the brightness of the sunlight?

Then be aware of your breath. Slow it down, if possible. Bring it down into your belly. Then just notice it without judgment.

Observe your thoughts. Is your mind chattering away or has it settled down to a more peaceful state? What about your emotions? Are you feeling happy? Sad? Perplexed?

Take in your surroundings. Tuning into your senses, what do you see? Hear? Feel? Smell? Taste?

Are you able to notice your inner experience (thoughts and feelings) while also paying attention to your outer experience? Coming into balance with the internal and external takes you to a state of peacefulness and calm.

Enjoy your walk and the inner stillness for as long as you want.

Gazing

Although many meditative practices use the breath as the focus, gazing uses a different focal point that will naturally slow down your breathing. Gazing is like staring at an object. To start, you'll probably want to select something in nature such as the following

the sky, or the clouds in the sky

gently lapping waves in the sea

a rock in a stream

the space between the leaves in a tree

a tree branch or cactus (for desert-dwellers like me)

a flower

a campfire

Once you have settled on the item, get into a comfortable position and look at it. Make whatever you have chosen the object of your attention.

Keep your eyes gently focused on it. Allow your eyes to remain soft and receptive. As you do this, the breath usually slows down and your thoughts become less and less distracting.

When you notice yourself being caught up in thoughts or aware of external movements or sounds, just calmly—without judgment—bring your attention back to the object.

When you are ready to end, softly close your eyes and take a few deep breaths. Feel yourself back in your body, feel the earth or floor beneath you, and then slowly open your eyes.

This meditative practice of gazing can shift your awareness, quiet your mind, and heighten your energy. In the stillness, you become more centered, peaceful, and calm. Sometimes when I do this gazing meditation, the object I am focusing on seems to move. And often whatever I am looking at appears to be outlined with white light.

Assignment

Pray and meditate. Begin and end each day in prayer, using a prayer that is significant to you or making one up with words from your heart. It can be as simple as "Good morning/Good night, Higher Power. Thank you for this day." Or combine a prayer of thanksgiving with a prayer of petition, or maybe a prayer for others as well as for yourself. It's up to you. The important part is your linking in with Spirit every morning and every night to deepen your spiritual connection.

◆

Stress is rampant in our modern lives, and meditation is an awesome stress-management technique and a superb tool to alleviate the anxiety that often leads to the first compulsive bite. You can feel the relaxation effect by practicing meditation just ten or fifteen minutes a day (setting a timer if you want). Meditating twice a day, when possible, is optimal. Do a conscious breathing meditation, walking meditation, gazing, or any meditation of your choosing every day—at least once a day. Try different types of meditation to find the ones that work best for you.

Day ⑨ Creative Visualization

As I began doing my own personal-growth work, I learned about the mind-body-spirit connection as a key component to optimal health. Whenever I explain this mind-body-spirit connection to clients, I like to start with a simple visualization: Imagine that you have a big, juicy, yellow lemon in your hand. Pretend that you have just been given a very sharp knife. Slice the lemon in half. See the juice oozing out onto the knife and cutting board. Now pick up half the lemon and take a bite. Yes, take a big bite. Imagine yourself chewing it.

As you cut and tasted the imaginary lemon, did you salivate? Most people do. How is it possible to pretend to have a lemon and have this kind of a reaction? This demonstrates how your thoughts move beyond your mind and can impact your body.

Creative visualization is a spiritual exercise using your thoughts and imagination to change your life in a positive way. Instead of thinking vaguely about your dreams and goals, you can visualize specific behaviors and events that you want to occur. Studies have shown that performances are enhanced for athletes and gymnasts when they go through a mental rehearsal imagining their entire routine in their minds before actually performing. During the visualizations, the neurons in your brain change to form new connections. Then, when you actively go through the experience, the brain cells are activated and recall what you have imagined, resulting in positive outcomes.

Fascinated with the possibilities this might hold, I eagerly read Shakti Gawain's book *Creative Visualization: Use the Power of Your Imagination to Create What You Want in Your Life*, as well as Adelaide Bry's *Visualization: Directing the Movies of Your Mind* and, later, Gerald Epstein's *Healing Visualizations: Creating Health Through Imagery* and Belleruth Naparstek's *Staying Well with Guided Imagery*. These books all confirm the notion that there is a definite mind-body-spirit connection for each of us. Our thoughts can affect our body and our health, and our thoughts can be impacted by how connected we feel to our spirit.

Creative visualization is a way to combine prayer and meditation. With prayer, you are putting forth your intentions to the Universe; with meditation, you are allowing the Universe to answer through images, sounds, or feelings.

Emotional eaters often have negative thoughts about their bodies, weight, eating behaviors, and themselves. The more you focus on the negative, the more you will continue to experience the negative in your life. By using creative visualization, you can set goals and use the power of your imagination to create what you want rather than what your negative thoughts might continue to bring you. Although it won't happen overnight and will involve work on your part, it is possible to use this tool to begin to design your new reality, one free from emotional eating.

Using the creative visualization technique is more concrete than daydreaming or just writing down your goals. When you do creative visualization, make sure you think in the first person (I), as if it were happening right now in the present time. Pay attention to as many senses as you can—concentrate and heighten each one. If you are unable to visualize a scene, focus on the feelings that arise as you imagine your intention has come true.

How about trying the following exercise right now to experience creative visualization for yourself?

Weight Loss Visualization

Imagine you're stepping on a scale after you have released some of your excess weight. Make it a realistic amount. If you have a hundred pounds to lose, see yourself on the scale with a twenty-pound weight loss. Or maybe a five-pound weight loss would thrill you. See yourself reacting to the weight loss with excitement, joy, and gratitude.

As you picture yourself on the scale, use all the senses you can to vividly create this image for yourself:

1. See the numbers on the scale. Make them large and clear so you can really see them.

2. Feel the excitement, the thrill. Where do you feel it in your body? Make it bigger, so you can really sense it.

3. Hear yourself making some whoopee noises or cheers or a big YES! Hear your internal voice congratulating yourself: I DID IT!

4. If there are any smells or tastes associated with this experience, heighten these also.

5. Again, feel the feelings—contentment, joy, exultation. Do your little happy dance!

Once you are really sensing the feelings and visualizing the scene you've created, imagine encasing it in a large pink bubble (a technique suggested by Shakti Gawain). Then let go of this beautiful pink bubble, sending it up into the air, watching it float up into the Universe, where it attracts the energy for manifestation.

◆

How did that feel? If this is a new experience for you, it might feel awkward and strange at first. With practice, it will become easier and easier. You have taken a goal (weight loss) and visualized it, created it, felt it, asked the Universe to give it to you, and then released it.

After reading books on creative visualization, I was convinced that this technique would work and eagerly tried it. My first attempt, however, didn't give me the immediate results I had expected. At the time I labeled myself a recovery consultant, and I was scheduled to teach an adult education class. I pictured myself excitedly presenting to a room full of people; I then enclosed the scene in a pink bubble and let it go. Confident that this technique would work, I was positive this would produce a standing-room-only audience. When I taught the class a week later, however, only four participants showed up!

Feeling disappointed that this tool I so much believed in didn't work, I forgot about creative visualization and the image I had placed in the pink bubble. A few months later, I taught the same class to a women's group. I never even thought of visualizing the size of my audience, but when I walked into the packed room, I was thrilled. It wasn't until the next day that I remembered the pink bubble imagery I had tried months earlier. And so it came to be—all in divine time. I came to understand that we can send our intention out into the Universe, but we can't control the timing of its manifestation.

What do you want to create that is within the realm of possibilities? Is there an event you'd like to happen? A behavior you want to incorporate? A reaction you'd like to change? For instance, let's say that every time your boss asks you to work late you get angry inside and reach for a candy bar or a handful of cookies to soothe yourself. In the creative visualization, you might want to see yourself with a different reaction (e.g., happy to be working overtime to earn extra money), or you might envision yourself finding an alternative to sweets for solace (e.g., deep, relaxing breathing).

Vision Boards

After successfully using creative visualizations for many years, I took it one step further and designed vision boards to have pictorial representations of my goals and dreams. Also called "treasure maps" or "dream boards," they are usually constructed as a collage of pictures, images, and affirmations (positive statements) to help clarify and maintain focus on a specific life goal. On my first vision board, for instance, one of my goals was to shed excess weight. I pasted a picture of a woman with a huge grin on her face as she stepped on the scale and another image of a woman wearing pants that had inches and inches of excess material because they were too large on her. As I looked at the vision board each morning, I said to myself, "This or something better, whatever is for the highest good."

Creative visualization takes place in the mind, and the vision board takes it one step further as a tangible representation of your intentions. Seeing it and energizing it each day helps you to stay positive as you envision the manifestation of your desires.

Assignment

The goal of this book is for you to have freedom from emotional eating. This means your relationship with food will change; it will no longer be your best friend or your worst enemy—food will be just food, used for pleasure, at times, and for nourishment. Being freed from emotional eating also means you are able to feel your feelings and deal with them rather than numbing yourself with food. Can you imagine yourself being free of the compulsive eating? Here are some steps to help you generate your own creative visualization:

See yourself as the person who is free from emotional eating with few cravings or urges. What does this look like? How are you relating to food? What do you do when you have big, uncomfortable emotions such as loneliness, fear, disappointment, or anger? Who are your support people? What is your relationship with your Higher Power? What positive messages are you telling yourself?

As you visualize yourself being free from emotional eating, bring in as many senses as you can, just as we did in the earlier scale example. Intensify all senses: Feel what you feel. See what you see. Hear what you hear. Smell what you smell. Taste what you taste.

Imagine placing the scene into a large pink bubble. Allow the bubble to float up into the sky toward the heavens. As it rises, you might want to say something like, "This or something better, whatever is for the highest good."

Perhaps you want to create a vision board using images from magazines, clip art, or your own albums. Look at your vision board every day. Stay positive. Visualize yourself handling feelings without reaching for food. Use these images as a meditation, if you want.

Imagine that you already have success and are no longer using food to deal with your emotions. How do you feel? How is your life better?

In this chapter, we focused on ourselves as spiritual beings and learned practices to deepen that spirituality and decrease the emotional eating. In the next chapter we discover ways to work with ourselves in a different area— as beings of energy.

Chapter 5

Energy Techniques

The next big frontier in medicine is energy medicine.
—Dr. Oz

HAVING EXPLORED MENTAL, EMOTIONAL, AND spiritual aspects of personal growth, we will now begin to take a look at energetic interventions and how they work together with those other techniques. Although I was trained in traditional talk therapy, I soon broadened my therapeutic skills as I investigated a new kind of healing treatment—energy medicine, also known as energy psychology or meridian therapy techniques. I learned that each of us is an energy being, and meridians—energy channels—run through our bodies (acupuncturists have known this for eons).

The term *energy* here refers to *subtle energy* or *vital life-force energy;* it is also known as *chi* (China), *ki* (Japan), *prana* (India), and *ankh* (ancient Egypt). For thousands of years, Eastern cultures, especially those from India and China, have taught that our bodies are made up of energy systems that influence our health and consciousness. We in the West have more recently been willing to incorporate energy practices for health. Energy psychology creatively combines ancient principles with new discoveries. These techniques influence the human energy system to release blocks and achieve balance.

According to Eastern medicine, all the pain, discomfort, and disease in the human body is the result of blocked energy flows. Following this theory, all our health problems, from the minor ones to the most serious, are caused by "stuck" energy. Sometimes known as "acupuncture without needles," meridian therapy techniques unblock energy, allowing it to flow more easily. And when you have no blockage or congestion, you have no pain. It's that simple. In addition to easing emotional and physical suffering, these breakthrough techniques can also mitigate food cravings and are an important adjunct for anyone with weight or body image issues.

Day ⑩ An Introduction to TFT and EFT

I've had the good fortune to study with many of the founders of the leading-edge techniques, including

- Francine Shapiro—EMDR (Eye Movement Desensitization and Reprocessing)
- Gary Craig—EFT (Emotional Freedom Techniques)
- Tapas Fleming—TAT (Tapas Acupressure Technique)
- Larry Nims—BSFF (Be Set Free Fast)

- Jim Durlacher—Acu-Power
- Donna Eden—Energy Medicine
- John Diepold—TAB (Touch and Breathe)
- Daniel Benor—WHEE (Whole Health Easily and Effectively, a hybrid derived from EMDR and EFT)

Meridian-based energy therapies often involve tapping on acupressure points. Why does tapping work? Dr. Dawson Church, author and researcher, discussed this question at a 2011 Tapping World Summit online event. When mental health professionals first used energy psychology techniques, many believed that the reason they worked is that they opened the body's energy flow, similar to how and why acupuncture works. This is true, but advanced research tells us there is even more involved. New experiences, thoughts, and emotions change our nervous system and brain very rapidly. Since trauma gets laid down very fast, why, Dr. Church reasoned, can't it be removed very quickly, too? We now know that the stress genes in our brains can get turned on within a second or two, and then our body produces adrenaline and cortisol. And cortisol can directly affect fat storage and weight gain, which means that stress helps make us fat.

Stress sends us into a fight-or-flight response, which was quite appropriate for our ancestors when a tiger was about to pounce. Nowadays, however, we have all kinds of stress, and our instinctual fight-or-flight response is overkill since we are not in physical danger. Tapping on acupressure points, Dr. Church believes, sends a calming signal to our body, giving our body the message that we are safe. As we tap, we release the upsetting feelings, relieve the stress, and feel better.

TFT

I first heard about Dr. Roger Callahan's TFT (Thought Field Therapy) through my friend and colleague Dr. Melanie Chimes. TFT involves tapping on specific points on the head and body to release emotional or physical pain. Melanie told me about it and I was very skeptical, thinking it looked and sounded absurd. My disparaging comment to her was "Thanks for the information, but I'm not interested in anything that weird."

A month later I co-facilitated a workshop around eliminating core beliefs. One participant, Bertha, had a distressing issue, and I worked with her using all the tools I knew, but she was not able to make a shift. Remembering that strange technique, TFT, which I didn't want to learn, I called Melanie. Over the phone, she led us through TFT, directing Bertha on what points to tap and what to say. Bertha's feelings cleared within minutes, and her challenging issue was suddenly no big deal. Skeptical Meryl became instantly ready to explore this innovative technology that had worked so fast with Bertha.

My colleagues and I hired a local teacher, Mary Stafford, and spent a day being trained in TFT. We learned that Dr. Callahan, a clinical psychologist in California who had studied Chinese medicine, the meridian system, and applied kinesiology (manual muscle testing), developed TFT out of his work with a woman named Mary. Mary had had such a severe phobia around water that she could only take a bath in a few inches of water, and she would not leave the house when it was raining. Although she had worked with Dr. Callahan for eighteen months, she'd made only minimal progress.

One day, Dr. Callahan decided to try something new: He asked Mary to think about water, and she felt intense anxiety. Then he muscle tested her and discovered a block in the stomach meridian. Knowing that the beginning of the stomach meridian is just below the eye (you can find it for yourself—feel the bone just below the center of each eye), he asked her to think about water while he gently tapped his fingers on this point.

Surprisingly, within just a few minutes, Mary announced the problem was gone and walked out of the house toward the swimming pool. Dr. Callahan, worried she might jump in and drown, shouted out, "Mary, don't go in! You can't swim." To which Mary yelled back, "The tapping took away my fear, Dr. Callahan—it didn't make me stupid!" Sure enough, Mary was able to go near the pool and even splash in the water with no fear. The terror plaguing Mary her entire life was gone, and it never returned.

EFT

Once I completed my training, I immediately began using TFT with my clients, with great success. Although I liked how fast it worked to eliminate emotional discomfort, I found the method cumbersome: I needed to have a cheat sheet nearby to remind me which points to tap for which feelings and in what order.

Then along came news of the work of Gary Craig, a Stanford-trained engineer who studied with Callahan and agreed that his technique worked. Gary streamlined the process by eliminating muscle testing and having us instead tap on all the suggested points. He developed EFT (Emotional Freedom Techniques), popularized this easy model, and made it accessible to mental health practitioners and the general public.

Fortunately, I was able to attend a seminar in Sedona, Arizona, to learn even more by studying with the founders of several of the energy modalities. Gary Craig trained the participants in additional EFT usages and led us through a few exercises. At one point, he had us each think of a fear and then do the tapping on ourselves. I was terrified of heights and hoped this would help. After a few rounds of tapping, I could picture myself on top of the Empire State Building without feeling any trepidation. I wondered, was my fear truly gone?

Soon enough, I had an opportunity to check it out. I went to Toronto to present at an energy psychology conference. While I was there, my colleagues and I took the glass elevator up the CN Tower, which at the time, was the world's tallest tower. Before getting on, I wondered if I'd be able to look down. During the one-minute ride to the top, I was delighted to be able to glance down with no fear. But the true test was coming: Could I stand on the observation deck, a thousand feet above the ground, and look down, without the old terror? I nervously stepped off the elevator and walked to the observation deck. I looked out. That was easy. Then, taking a big breath, I looked down—and was delighted to take in the landscape. The fear really was gone!

Gary's words to us after teaching EFT: "Try it on everything!" And so I did. I have dozens and dozens of stories to share. Attending a workshop a few weeks later, for example,

I heard the sobbing of a young teen while I was using the restroom. Remembering Gary's words, I approached her and said, "You are obviously in a lot of pain. I know a technique that might be helpful and involves tapping on acupressure points. Would you be interested in experiencing this?"

Her companion yelled out, "Do it, do it, do it. My friend does tapping with her therapist, and it's great."

The distraught teen agreed to experience the tapping technique, and I showed her the places to tap while repeating, "Feeling upset." Within a few minutes, the river of tears had stopped and her breathing had returned to normal. She told me that she was attending a leadership conference at the hotel and had just found out she lost the presidency by a few votes. The disappointment was so intense she could not stop crying. Once she completed a round of tapping, however, she hopped down from the sink where she had been sitting and calmly exited the restroom.

Now you might be wondering why I am spending so much time telling you about EFT. Simple. We eat when we have painful feelings. Using EFT and other energy techniques neutralizes the feelings so we no longer feel compelled to munch! So stay with me as I go through a few more examples.

I have also had great success using EFT to eliminate phobias. Living in Arizona, I encounter a lot of people who have fears and phobias around creepy, crawly things, especially snakes and scorpions. Since I have been very successful in helping folks eradicate their fears, I volunteered to demonstrate my work with overcoming snake phobias for a television newscast in Tucson. Patty was so scared of snakes that she sprinted from her house to the car each morning, and she was terrified when she was out walking her dog. Her husband enjoyed gentle hiking, but she refused to go because she might see a snake. And, to her husband's chagrin, she dreamed of snakes almost every night and ferociously kicked him in bed as they were sleeping. Both Patty and her husband wanted to cure this phobia.

I met the two of them at their home and did a few rounds of tapping with Patty. Her fear was lessened immensely, and we decided to meet at a reptile store the next day. Before entering the store, I did one more round of tapping on Patty. Then she strolled into the store and, to her surprise, enjoyed looking at the snakes within their glass enclosures, even expressing wonderment at how beautiful they were. The store owner removed one snake and held it, stroking it and saying it felt soft. I asked Patty if she wanted to touch it, and she pulled back. Then, much to our amazement, she walked over, touched the snake, and exclaimed, "It is soft!" Overwhelmed with relief, she burst into tears. A few weeks later, I learned she and her husband were now able to enjoy walking their dog and hiking Sabino Canyon with no fear of snakes. You can check out the news clip at *www.tinyurl.com/merylfearofsnakes*.

As emotional eaters, we all reach for food when the big feelings hit. EFT is an easy-to-use tool to utilize instead. Without our big feelings, would we need to stuff our faces? What fears or anxieties do you have? Sometimes you can clear these yourself using EFT. Other times, it is best to seek the support of a trained practitioner.

Let's get started using EFT. You will be tapping acupressure points mostly on the head and upper body using your fingertips of one or (preferably) both hands. Tap lightly (when I first learned this, I tapped too hard and ended up with some bruises!) but solidly.

EFT Directions

Step 1: Begin by thinking of a time when you had a big feeling and you compulsively overate. Identify the feeling or feelings you are having at this moment (not how you felt at the time). Are you feeling mad, sad, afraid, anxious, lonely, guilty, etc.?

Step 2: Rate the feeling. How intense is it right now? Use the scale of 0–10, with 0 being nothing and 10 being the most intense.

Step 3: Once you have identified and rated the feeling, start tapping on what's known as the Karate Chop Point—the edge of either hand between your wrist and little finger, and say aloud, "Even though I am feeling _____ [insert feeling], I deeply and completely accept myself." Some examples might be:

- "Even though I am feeling anxious, I deeply and completely accept myself."
- "Even though I am feeling lonely, I deeply and completely accept myself."
- "Even though I am in a funk, I deeply and completely accept myself."

(**Note:** If it is too big a leap for you to declare, "I deeply and completely accept myself," you can instead say, "I *want to* deeply and completely accept myself.")

Repeat this three times.

Step 4: After the Karate Chop Point, you will do a sequence of tappings, repeating a reminder phrase: "this _____ [insert feeling]." Tap on each of the points listed below five to seven times as you say the reminder phrase.

> **TH**—top of head (can move fingers around crown)
>
> **EB**—inside edge of eyebrow
>
> **SE**—side of eye
>
> **UE**—under eye (the stomach meridian point mentioned earlier)
>
> **UN**—under nose
>
> **CH**—chin, right in the middle
>
> **CB**—just below collarbone, near breastbone
>
> **UA**—under arm (I have heard it said, "In line with the nipples for men and where they used to be for women!")
>
> **WR**—tap the insides of your wrists together

Step 5: Reassess: Take a breath. Think of the original incident. What is the intensity of your feeling now? If you are at a 0 or 1, you have discharged the feeling. If you are higher than a 1, repeat the process.

EFT can feel a bit strange at first, but it gets easier with practice.

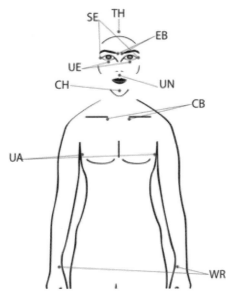

Assignment

In chapter 2 you started a food-mood diary. Take a look at it now, and notice your patterns. What feelings are consistently present when you overeat? You now have a personal intervention tool at your disposal to get rid of those yucky feelings so you won't have to numb out with food.

Perform EFT on yourself. Think of a time when you had a big feeling and you compulsively overate. You might choose something that you wrote about in your food-mood diary, or maybe there is something happening right now that causes you emotional discomfort when you think about it. Is there a situation that usually sends you in search of something sweet? Maybe your child is not listening, and you feel frustrated. Is there something that happened in the past that still vexes you? Maybe you ate too much yesterday, and you are angry with yourself. Pick one specific incident, think about it, and allow yourself to feel the feelings you are having right now—not the feelings you had yesterday—as you remember it. Rate that feeling on a scale of 0–10. Start with the Karate Chop Point, and move through the sequence of points as explained above. How intense is the feeling once you've finished? If it is higher than a 1, do additional rounds of tapping until you've reduced the intensity down to a 0 or 1.

EFT is a great tool for releasing uncomfortable feelings. Otherwise, we might do what we have done so often in the past—eat over them. As human beings, we do whatever we can to avoid pain, so learning to use food to numb the feelings was a beneficial coping skill when we were children. Now that we are adults, however, we have healthier options. Sometimes we need to feel the feelings in order to work with them. Other times, though, the tapping techniques help us clear the overwhelming emotions so we won't need to stuff them with food.

Day (11) Rapidly Integrated Transformation Technique (RITT)

After learning EFT and other energy modalities, my colleague Robin Trainor Masci and I developed an offshoot technique called Rapidly Integrated Transformation Technique (RITT). It is based particularly on Larry Nims's Be Set Free Fast, which includes clearing the roots of the feelings, and John Diepold's Touch and Breathe. Most of our clients are involved in Twelve-Step Programs, and although they liked EFT, they wanted a technique that included a spiritual component as well, and RITT does that. I have successfully used both EFT and RITT to help clients with eating issues, and I have taught energy techniques to mental health professionals who have also had much success. Many have said they choose EFT when there is one predominant feeling and RITT when there are several big feelings at once.

The main difference between EFT and RITT is that EFT repeats the same reminder phrase throughout (such as *this anger*), and RITT uses a script that mentions numerous feelings. The points we tap on with RITT are the same that you learned for EFT, with a few exceptions: The Side of Eye Point (SE) is not used in RITT, and the Third Eye Point (in between the eyebrows) has been added, as have some spots on the fingers. In addition, the Heart Point is added (it is sometimes used in EFT but was not mentioned earlier, because it is not always used). If possible, use both sides of your body for the Eyebrow, Under Eye, Collarbone, and Under Arm Points for maximum results.

Rapidly Integrated Transformation Technique (RITT)

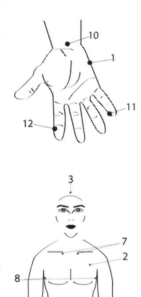

Basic Directions: Think of an issue, and note your level of discomfort (0 = none, 10 = intense). Or think of a craving, and note your level of desire (0 = no urge, 10 = intense urge).

Imagine you are a tree and will be clearing from the branches (the conscious mind) to the roots (the sub-conscious). As you lightly tap each point using two or three fingers, think about the issue or craving and read aloud what is in quotation marks below.

◆

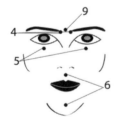

1. Karate Chop Point— tap outside edge of hand

   Say: "I release this issue [or challenge or craving] to my Higher Power/God/Spirit to transform it and my relationship to it, never to take it back again or passively receive it back."

2. Heart Point (spot above left breast where your hand goes for the Pledge of Allegiance)—gently rub in a circle toward shoulder.

   Say three times: "Even though I have this issue, I totally and completely love and accept myself."

3. Crown (top of head)—tap around in a circle

   Say: "I bring Higher Power/Spirit/God/Light into all the branches to the deepest roots around this issue and ask for healing for the highest good."

4. Eyebrow—tap where the eyebrows start, near bridge of nose

   Say: "I release all the sadness in all the branches to the deepest roots around this issue."

5. Under Eye—tap on bone just under the center of each eye

   Say: "I release all the fear in all the branches to the deepest roots around this issue."

6. Chin and Under Nose—tap both spots at once

   Say: "I release all the shame and all the embarrassment in all the branches to the deepest roots around this issue."

7. Collarbone—tap two finger widths beneath inside of collarbones (close to breastbone)

   Say: "I release all the hurt and all the grief in all the branches to the deepest roots around this issue."

8. Under Arm—tap spot about four inches below armpit, in line with nipple

   Say: "I release all the guilt in all the branches to the deepest roots around this issue."

9. Third Eye Point—tap between eyebrows

   Say: "I release all the trauma in all the branches to the deepest roots around this issue."

10. Inside Wrist—tap where watchband would fasten, palm side of wrist

Say: "I release all the pain in all the branches to the deepest roots around this issue."

11. Little Finger (either hand)—tap on the side nearest the ring finger next to the nail

Say: "I release all the anger in all the branches to the deepest roots around this issue."

12. Index Finger—tap the side nearest the thumb next to the nail

Say at least three of the following:

- "I release all the energy invested in this issue so I can use that energy for my own well-being."

- "I totally and completely forgive myself for forgetting that I am doing the best can."

- "I totally and completely forgive myself for allowing this issue to disturb my peace of mind."

- "I totally and completely forgive myself, and I intend to forgive everyone else involved."

- "I totally and completely forgive myself, and I ask for the wisdom to see that everyone involved was acting from a place of unmet needs."

Breathe. Reassess your level of discomfort or level of urge. If above 1, repeat steps 1–12. When at 0 or 1, continue to step 13.

13. Repeat steps 4 (Eyebrow) through 11 (Little Finger)

Say at each point: "I bring in Higher Power/Spirit/God/Light to replace the _____ [sadness, etc.] in all the branches to the deepest roots around this issue."

Assignment

We're going to use an expanded version of RITT today, adjusted for cravings. To start, you'll need a food item that calls you, such as chips or candy, so go and get it now. For this exercise, you will need the actual substance in front of you. When Gary Craig introduced a similar exercise using EFT, he handed out Hershey's Kisses. Please use whatever item you might be craving, though to simplify it, I refer to chocolate kisses as we go through the exercise.

Before you proceed, it is important to assess your level of craving, with 0 indicating no urge whatsoever and 10 indicating the most intense craving. Write your number down on a piece of paper. Next, unwrap the kiss, hold it to your nose and smell it, and then take a tiny taste. Did the intensity of the craving increase? If so, write down the new number (10 is high).

Now, with the kiss in front of you, do the following:

1. Tap the Karate Chop Point (the edge of either hand between the little finger and the wrist), with two or three fingers of the other hand and repeat the following words: "I release this craving to God/Spirit/ Higher Power/Universe to transform it and my relationship to it, never to take it back again or passively receive it back."

2. Find the Heart Point—a lymph drainage spot on the left side of your chest, approximately where you would place your hand if pledging allegiance. It is known as "the sore spot" because it often feels tender

when you poke at it. [Note, if you wear a pacemaker, use the right side of your chest.] Gently rub this area in a circular motion while saying "Even though I have this craving, I totally and completely accept myself." Repeat. On the third time change it to "Even though I have this craving, I am ready to release it now."

3. Tapping the crown of your head, say, "I bring God/ Spirit/Higher Power/Universe into all the branches to the deepest roots around this craving." Take a deep breath in and out.

4. Tapping the inside corner of both eyebrows, say, "I release all the sadness in all the branches to the deepest roots around this craving." Holding your fingers on the spots, take a deep breath. Imagine releasing the feelings as the breath goes out.

5. Tapping the bone or notch in the bone just beneath the center of each eye, say, "I release all the fear in all the branches to the deepest roots around this craving." Take a breath with fingers still touching the points and exhale out the fear.

6. Using the sides of your index finger and thumb, tap just below the nose and just below the lip, saying, "I release all the shame and all the embarrassment in all the branches to the deepest roots around this craving." Hold the hand still on the points and take a deep breath, releasing the feelings as you breathe out.

7. Tapping two finger widths beneath the inside of the collarbones, say, "I release all the hurt

and all the grief in all the branches to the deepest roots around this craving." Hold the points and breathe, letting the feelings go as you let go of the breath.

8. Tapping the under arm points, say, "I release all the guilt in all the branches to the deepest roots around this craving." Holding your hands still, take a deep breath as you exhale the feelings.

9. Tapping between the eyebrows, the Third Eye Point, say, "I release all the trauma in all the branches to the deepest roots around this craving." Holding the point, take another breath, releasing the feelings on the exhale.

10. Tapping the insides of the wrists together, say, "I release all the pain in all the branches to the deepest roots around this craving." Holding the insides of the wrists together, take another deep breath, letting go of the feelings as you breathe out.

11. Tapping the inside edge of the little finger on either hand (next to the nail bed), say, "I release all the anger in all the branches to the deepest roots around this craving." Hold the point. Breathe. Exhale out the anger.

12. Tapping the edge of the index finger (the edge closest to the thumb) next to the nail bed, say,

   • "I release all the energy invested in this issue so I can use the energy for my own well-being."

- "I totally and completely forgive myself for forgetting I am doing the best I can."
- "I totally and completely forgive myself for having this craving."
- "I totally and completely love and accept myself, even though I eat for emotional reasons."
- "I totally and completely love and accept myself, and I am ready to release this craving now."

Take another deep breath and then reassess. Pick up the chocolate kiss, smell it, taste it. What is your level of craving now? Did it go down? If not, or if it is not yet at a 0 or 1, then go through the script again.

Once I learned energy psychology techniques, I went back through my personal history to find all memories with a negative charge. Then I would think of the incident as I tapped until there were no longer uncomfortable feelings connected with the memory. Although I had already done a lot of personal work on myself, I was amazed to find so many negatively-charged memories, and even more amazed to see how fast the discomfort abated because of the tapping. I continue to use EFT and RITT every opportunity I have: When I walk past the freezer and the ice cream shouts, "I'm here for you!" or when I have an urge for something sweet, I can choose to tap to eliminate the craving. When I am feeling angry, sad, lonely, afraid, ashamed, or hurt, I tap. When I want to celebrate or reward myself by going to food, I tap. Sometimes I still do the actual tapping on my head and body points; other times I just imagine tapping the points. Yes, that's right. Once your body has had some experiences with the tapping, then just thinking about tapping on the points will bring about the same result! This is the mind-body connection that we explored on Day 9 (remember the lemon?).

Tapping is one of the most useful tools you can have to deal directly with cravings and emotional discomfort. When you remember to tap, you will eat by choice rather than by compulsion.

Day (12) Personal Energy Work

As compulsive eaters, when our energy is low, we often turn to food as a quick pick-me-up. Sometimes food grounds us, sometimes it invigorates us, and sometimes it just reinforces a habit—that of reaching for something to chew on. Let's now take a look at alternatives to help us feel revived and energized.

When introducing the concept of personal life-force energy to my clients, I often guide them through the following exercise. Try it now, if you like, or later, as part of your assignment for today.

Sending Energy Exercise

Sitting in a comfortable position with your spine straight, allow your tongue to rest behind your top front teeth. Tune into your breath as you breathe in and breathe out. Don't change it—just be aware of it. Does your belly rise with the inhale? Do you feel the air moving in and out of your lungs? Become conscious of your breath.

Now, imagine a large bright light just above your head. As you inhale, visualize bringing the light in through the top of your head and down into your heart. Exhale. Breathe in again, allowing the light/energy to flow into your heart; breathe out and send this light/energy to all the cells in your body. Do it yet again: Inhale, filling your heart with this energy and light from above. Exhale, this time sending it out to any part of your body that is tight or achy or in pain. Repeat five to ten times.

Next, imagine a brilliant white light in the earth just beneath you. This time, bring the light and energy up through your feet or up through your tailbone into your heart as you inhale. Exhale. Again, breathe in and bring the earth energy up through your tailbone or feet and into your heart. Exhale and send the light/energy to all your internal organs. Repeat five to ten times.

Now, if you are able, combine the two: When you inhale, bring in the light from above through your crown down into your heart, and at the same time, bring the earth energy up through your tailbone or feet into your heart. Exhale and send this light/energy out into the Universe, to wherever it is needed. Try it again. Bring the light and energy into your heart simultaneously from the earth and from the heavens; exhale it out to specific people or places, wherever it is needed. Repeat five to ten times.

◆

Feeling more relaxed? More energized? More centered? Perhaps you feel tingly. Those are the usual responses after doing this exercise. This is great to do whenever you want more energy or if you desire to feel more centered and calm. You can use this exercise to send energy to parts of your own body that are in pain, stressed, or tight. And you can also use this technique to send energy to other people.

We are all energy beings and we have a battery pack of energy. We need to keep our personal battery pack charged or we will feel drained and reach for that first compulsive bite. Exercises like this help us keep our batteries fully charged. Have you ever noticed that you feel tired and drained after spending time with a certain person? Maybe that person is ill, or depressed, or stressed out. Often, when we are with people whose energy is lower than ours, we can feel depleted, and more prone to grab something to eat.

So what can we do to keep our energy from being drained? The simplest thing is to do the Sending Energy Exercise described above and send the person Source energy, which is in infinite supply. When you bring in the energy of the Universe, you are not sending your personal energy—you are sending Universal or Source energy. It is extremely important to not send your own energy, for you have a finite amount and you can easily become drained.

But the energy from Source is infinite, and you can tap into it whenever you want.

Sending someone energy is a win-win: Whenever you channel Universal energy to anyone, your own body takes what it needs first and then sends it on. As you energize the other, you become energized yourself. Sending energy often changes the person and can even change the relationship between the two of you.

For example, Robin and I used to facilitate a monthly workshop in Cleveland, Ohio. At the beginning of each session, everyone would check in, sharing feelings and breakthroughs since the last time we were together. One of the participants, Sam, talked about hating his boss. Sam is a recovering alcoholic and goes to AA meetings. His boss, however, was an untreated alcoholic and caused Sam a lot of grief on the job. Sam hated going to work and told us he didn't know how much longer he could take it because his boss was such a jerk.

We suggested that Sam send energy (using the preceding exercise) to his boss. Sam was adamant: "I am not going to send that SOB energy." I reminded Sam that he should not send his own energy under any circumstances, but he could send Universal energy to his employer. Sam wasn't sure he was up to the task.

The following month Sam attended the workshop again, and when it was his turn to check in, he talked about his boss. This time, however, he expressed a different viewpoint: "I used to think my boss was a jerk, but we went for coffee and talked and now he goes to AA meetings with me. He's really a good guy!"

What changed? I could hardly wait to ask, and when I did, Sam declared, "Oh, I forgot to tell you. Last month when I was here, it was suggested I send energy to my boss. I was resistant and didn't want to at all. I mean, I didn't like the guy—why would I want to send him energy? But one day at work when he was driving me crazy, I decided to try it. I called in energy from above and sent it through my heart, directing it to him. I did it again the next day and the next. On the fourth day, he asked if I wanted to have coffee, and he confided in me that he had a booze problem. I invited him to go to an AA meeting with me, and he went again the following week. He's really a good guy, and I can't believe the difference in our relationship!"

Sending energy often improves the connection between two people, it costs nothing, and it feels good for both the sender and the receiver.

My daughter knows this technique of getting energized and so do her children. In fact, it is not unusual for the kids to suggest we send energy to their mom when she is tired. As soon as we start, my daughter begins to giggle and often yells out, "Stop. Enough. The last time you did this I couldn't sleep." High energy for her (and for me) often results in giggling and sometimes even hysterical, contagious laughter.

When you get to the Assignment portion of this day, you will try it for yourself. Remember, this is not your own energy. This is energy from the Universe, and it is limitless. Although it goes through your heart, remember, *it is not your energy.*

Before I understood energy, whenever I had a session with a depressed or low-energy client, I felt drained and had trouble staying awake. Not wanting to nod off during the session, I would surreptitiously dig my fingernails into my other palm in an effort to stay present. At that time, I didn't know that these low-energy clients, at an unconscious level, were drawing on my energy to feel better themselves. This is not done maliciously. The people who pull on your energy or feed off of you are sometimes known as energy vampires. Since there is no harmful intent, I prefer to just refer to them as folks with low energy.

In addition to clients, I have had plenty of other experiences with low-energy people and its ramifications. A relative came to visit me in Tucson. She tends to be low energy, so she loves being with me because she always feels better in my presence. Once I understood more about how energy works, I knew how important it was for me to continue sending it to her when we were together so she would not be drawing on my energy at an unconscious level. She stayed with me for a few days, and she felt great and I felt great—I was remembering to send or channel energy to her. The last day, I got up early to take her to the airport, and I returned home too tired to take my morning walk. Instead, I lay down on the couch and slept for a few hours. I wasn't sure why I was so exhausted until I remembered the energy work. Or, to be more accurate, the lack of it! The days she was visiting, I was conscious about sending her energy. The morning she left, however, I got up early, drove her to the airport, and did not remember to send energy to her. So she took from me instead, and I felt drained. It was a great reminder that it is imperative to stay conscious when you're with low-energy people, remembering to be in channel mode—bring in the energy from Source, through the heart, to the other person, so both of you feel invigorated.

Begin to monitor your energy level throughout the day, and pay attention to what kinds of people, things, and activities give you energy, and what drains you. When you are low energy, there is a tendency to reach for food for a boost. Gathering a wide array of tools to combat fatigue and low energy offers you other options.

One of the best ways you can increase your energy and vitality is to reduce the amount or the effects of destructive stress. Tapping techniques can be beneficial, and so can breathing techniques and meditation. Walking and other exercise also decrease the effects of stress. What are your favorite stress reducers? Keep several ideas on hand in your toolbox so that stress doesn't push you into emotional eating in an attempt to feel better.

When you do today's assignment, you will have a chance to write your own lists of energizers and drains. Below is a list of several of mine:

Energizers: Being with my granddaughters, doing energy work such as EFT and RITT, channeling or sending energy to others or to myself, having happy thoughts, walking in nature, playing with my dog or cats, writing a gratitude list, letting go of resentments, being with certain people (especially high-energy people and people who I know love me), being in the ocean, smelling a fragrant rose, snorkeling, dancing, being in joy, meditating, doing breath work, feeling connected to God and to the angels, teaching, singing, laughing, looking into the eyes of a newborn baby, and doing healing work.

Energy Drains: Being with low-energy people (sick, depressed) or people caught up in their dramas, illness, difficult emotions (lots of feelings are energy drains; it is important to feel the feeling and then discharge it—by expressing it or tapping or journaling), being overtired, feeling too responsible for too many things, feeling a time crunch, feeling overwhelmed, having unmet expectations, overworking, and not getting enough sleep.

Make sure you begin to identify both your energizers and your drains. When you need a shot of energy, open your energizer list and pick an item that you can do right then to revitalize yourself.

Energy Pick-Me-Ups

Here are some pick-me-ups you can use rather than reaching for a sugary treat or an energy drink when you need an energy boost:

- Stand up. Allow your arms to make large figure eights. Great. Now switch and go in the other direction. As you move your arms through the air, you are increasing your energy field, and you should be feeling more energized.

- Think of something that brings you joy. Imagine this joy moving through your body, into all your cells. Breathe in the joy.

Stop Eating Your Heart Out

- Laughter is very energizing. Repeat the syllables: "Ho ho he he ha ha." Say it again and again until you are laughing out loud.

- Clap your hands. Stand and give yourself applause. It is nice if someone else can do it for you; if not, do it for yourself.

- March in place—pick up those legs and swing your arms. Large muscle movement helps diminish stress and increases the flow of energy.

- Tapping two finger widths beneath your collarbones (known as the K-27 points by acupuncturists) can help you feel more energized. Cross your hands over each other if that's comfortable for you. Take some nice breaths as you tap.

- Do the Cross Crawl: Stand up. Touch your right hand to your left knee and then your left hand to your right knee. You can lift your knees to meet your hands if you want. Repeat ten times or so.

- Go outside. Absorb some vitamin D from the sunlight. Take a few deep breaths in the fresh air.

- Here's a simple one that often works: Drink a glass of water!

Becoming aware of your energy drains will give you the opportunity to change, modify, or eliminate many of them. For instance, if you are planning to be with someone who is low energy, you can send or channel energy while you're with that person. Actually, you can start even before seeing the person—as you think of the individual, imagine sending energy, and the person (though unaware) will receive it.

Drama is a huge energy drain for everyone—I'm referring here to the way a person overreacts or exaggerates the significance of mild events and does so for attention or to spice up life. I am sure you have heard the term *drama queen*. Can you hear a friend's tale of woe and stay in the place of observer and not get pulled in? It would be to your advantage to try this. The next time someone tells you all the awful stuff that's going on, stay neutral and give empathy without getting sucked into the energy of the story. Here is the difference in responses: "Oh, you poor thing. How awful. They should be punished for that," means you are probably caught up in the drama of it all. On the other hand, "That is really hard for you, how can I support you?" probably indicates that you have stayed out of the drama and are in the position of observer or supportive friend.

What about other energy drains? Fluorescent lights seem to bother a lot of people. If this is a drain for you, limit the amount of time you are under those lights as much as you can. If that isn't possible, do energy practices while those lights are shining on you. Illness is hard to work with except by doing the obvious—do what you need to do to restore your health: Rest; drink plenty of water; stay positive. Feelings, too, can be a big drain on your energy—especially unexpressed feelings. When I think back to my childhood with all the unspoken, pushed-down feelings, I am not surprised I suffered from childhood depression. Think of the feelings that bring you down—sadness, grief, loneliness, etc. If we look at the world and believe there is a Divine Plan, then when we are in the midst of uncomfortable feelings, we can say to ourselves, "This too shall pass." Using meridian therapies to clear distressing feelings is one of the quickest ways to release emotional discomfort and return to building your energy.

Assignment

Personal energy work begins with monitoring your energy and discovering your energizers and drains. Write out a list of energizers and one of drains, and include whatever gives or depletes your energy. When you feel low, pick an energizer or two from the list rather than reaching for something to munch. Be aware of the energy drains so you're not blindsided by them.

Assess your energy right now using a 0–10 scale with 10 being high. If you are below a 7, do one or more of the quick-energy pick-me-ups described above or one of the energizers from your own list. Reassess your energy level. Still too low? Continue trying other energizers until your energy is a 7 or higher and you feel enlivened. Get in the habit of monitoring your energy level and taking steps to build it before it dips too low. The lower your energy, the easier it is to succumb to emotional eating; the higher your energy, the easier it is to just eat for physical hunger.

Practice sending energy. Once you are comfortable with it, you can use it any time you are in a difficult situation or with challenging people, rather than having the people or situation push you into compulsive eating behaviors. You can send energy to yourself, to another person, or to a part of your own body, and you'll feel energized just doing it.

Chapter 6

Going Within
. . . .

*By choosing not to allow parts of ourselves to exist,
we are forced to expend huge amounts of psychic
energy to keep them beneath the surface.*
—DEBBIE FORD, *THE DARK SIDE OF THE LIGHT CHASERS*

YOU HAVE BEEN BUILDING NEW skills, and achieving a new
level of self-awareness as you completed the past twelve
days' assignments. This kind of life-enhancing personal-
growth work can be both exciting and scary. It includes
the process of discovering disowned parts of the self, making peace with yourself, and becoming the best you that
you can be. It is a journey to wholeness. This chapter continues this exploration and provides you an opportunity to
go to previously unexplored realms within yourself.

When you get a splinter, it needs to be removed completely. If you ignore it or don't pull it out entirely, the skin
could grow over the foreign body and hide it from view so
it would look okay. But looks can be deceiving, and the
wound might be festering beneath the skin, causing pain

when the area is touched. Even though you don't see the irritant deeply embedded under many layers of skin, for the sake of your health, it must be extracted. Likewise, traumas can be smoldering under the surface and need to be healed.

As kids, we face many lowercase-*t* traumas such as being humiliated, hearing our parents fighting, or having a friend move away. Some children have also endured capital-*T* Traumas—divorce, family deaths, abuse, accidents, or major illnesses. As adults, we carry internal scars connected to unresolved issues from childhood traumas, often at the unconscious or subconscious level. Just because they are below the surface doesn't mean we are not impacted by them. Look at how we use food for emotional reasons—possibly an indication of unresolved trauma from the past.

As you think back on your childhood, you might not remember any lowercase-*t* traumas or even capital-*T* Traumas. Alice Miller, in her book *For Your Own Good: Hidden Cruelty in Child-Rearing and the Roots of Violence*, contends that people—possibly hiding traumatic events from their own consciousness—often defend their parents' childrearing practices, saying something like "Even though I was hit, it was for my own good." Her website tells us "For a child to develop naturally, it needs respect from its caregivers, tolerance for its feelings, awareness of its needs and sensibilities, and authenticity on the part of its parents." Many (most?) of us overeaters didn't get that.

The Ten Commandments are very clear that we must respect our parents. But is it taught anywhere that parents should respect their children?

Babies are born into an imperfect world with imperfect parents. Although the offspring are (usually) very loved and wanted, the new mothers and fathers come to the task of parenting with their own baggage—challenges, wounds, personality quirks, insecurities, their own unhealed traumas, and more. Watching folks deal with their children in public places, I find it astounding that so many of us turn out as seemingly well as we do! No decent parent gets up each morning thinking, *What can I do today to screw up my kid?* But we have not evolved enough yet as a human race to not hurt our children, and even the most loving of parents may inflict cruelty on their children without conscious intention.

In addition, as children, we often come to erroneous conclusions about ourselves based on our caregivers' words and actions. Up to around six years of age, we have no cognitive conscious filters in place to interpret the information we absorb from our environment. Therefore, as little kids, we make up stories in our own minds about what is happening to us or around us, and that becomes our truth.

If you know your parents were tyrannical and you faced many traumas or Traumas, then there is work to do to heal the emotional scars, and it would serve you to consult a trauma professional. If your memories are mostly about loving, caring parents, and you are reading this book because you use and abuse food as if it were a drug, then you may have to dig for the splinter that's hidden from your conscious awareness. Unhealed trauma accompanied by suppressed emotions can be the engine driving your food compulsion.

When I first started going to Twelve-Step meetings at the age of twenty-nine, I listened intently to the stories being told by one member after another about being raised in a dysfunctional family. I felt sorry for these people, and I thought to myself, *It's too bad they had such a hard time. My family wasn't dysfunctional—I had an idyllic childhood.* But when I stopped the compulsive overeating, memories and feelings began to emerge that I had no idea were even there. I knew my parents loved me, but I also had to admit that my childhood was not perfect and that I was harboring a lot of resentments and old wounds. Employing the methods set forth throughout this book—and especially this chapter—I dug out some putrefying splinters and began to heal the unresolved traumas and squelched feelings.

Day (13) The Inner Child

Earlier, I mentioned that journaling was very important in my recovery. As I spent many hours writing, old (seemingly forgotten) memories began to wiggle loose and move into my conscious mind. I had no problem remembering that I felt sad and abandoned when I was four and my father became a traveling salesman—I missed my daddy and couldn't understand why he was gone all week. As I went deeper into this memory, I uncovered the story I told myself around it—my four-year-old little being concluded, *If I were enough, he wouldn't leave me.* Thus, my identity of being not-enough was forged and became an integral part of how I perceived myself for many years.

When people are feeling whole and good about themselves, they attract others who complement this conviction.

The opposite is also true: When people believe they are inadequate, they magnetize people and situations that continue to mirror back to them ways they are deficient. Believing that I was defective, I began wearing an invisible sign announcing to the world *I Am Not Enough*, which drew people and experiences to me that continued to validate my truth, that I was inferior and worthless.

Somewhere along the way in Twelve-Step Recovery, I learned about Inner Child work. Charles Whitfield, in his book *Healing the Child Within*, defines the Child Within (his term for the Inner Child) as "that part of each of us which is ultimately alive, energetic, creative and fulfilled; it is our real self—who we truly are." The Inner Child can be seen as a metaphor for the precious child we all were, who often had unexpressed feelings and unmet needs. Working with this Child Within helps uncover and then heal old childhood wounds so they no longer impact you as an adult.

In the past, you have used food, and other means, to not have to look at disturbing memories from days gone by. These (often) submerged memories exist, however, and need to be brought to the surface just like that old infected splinter that needs removing. Otherwise, events in the present can continue to trigger the past, and you may find yourself overreacting and wondering why you are so bothered by something that is seemingly trivial. Start to become aware of this for yourself: When you have a big adverse reaction to a person, place, or event, it is often an indication that your young part, your Inner Child, needs some healing around it. The past is not just the past—it invades the present, and, like the unwelcome intruder it can be, it might bring conflict, despair, and other big feelings out of proportion to the triggering event.

Becoming aware of the Child Within and getting to know that forever-young part of you begins to free you from the shackles of the past and encourages you to enjoy the happy, spontaneous Wonder Child part of yourself. The Inner Child can be an infant, a toddler, or even a rebellious adolescent. It is alive within you. It needs you and is

- playful and curious,
- the innocent part of yourself that needs protection,
- the scared, hurt part that keeps emotions pushed away,
- the vulnerable part that needs nurturance and love,
- that part of your psyche that retains the feelings you experienced as a child,
- embedded in your emotional body or subconscious,
- waiting for the Healthy Adult part of you to give the child part a voice.

When I learned to do Inner Child work, my goal was re-parenting the young child in me who had achieved excellence in beating herself up. She believed she was not good enough and desperately needed a nurturing parent who would unconditionally love her and gently show her where her perceptions might be skewed. I stepped up and took on that role. Doing Inner Child work revealed to me the immense amount of pain I felt as a youngster, as well as to the awful things I said to myself and thought about myself. I learned to listen, and I learned to give empathy, compassion, and unconditional love to my younger self.

It is important, whenever doing Inner Child work, to always take the role of the Nurturing Parent or Healthy Adult. The child already has heard enough criticism from the outside—parents, friends, community, clergy, teachers—and also from the Inner Critic. When there is a Healthy Adult present, the young part begins to trust and open up. If, when doing this work, the Critical Parent shows up and uses a harsh voice to respond to the young part, the child becomes re-traumatized and will clam up.

Getting in touch with the Child Within can be rewarding, comforting, and healing. It can also be upsetting whenever the Inner Child tells you about past hurts and pain. When this happens, many people want to discontinue working with the Child Within. If you want to heal, I beseech you to stay in the place of the Healthy Adult and listen to the child's pain to allow the healing to happen. If this is too much for you, consider doing this work with a trauma specialist. Just giving voice to the old hurts and hearing a compassionate response is sometimes enough to heal.

A significant book for me was John Bradshaw's *Healing the Shame That Binds You*. In it, he says,

> It is important to note that the need to find the Inner Child is part of every human being's journey toward wholeness. No one had a perfect childhood. Everyone bears the unresolved unconscious issues of his family history (142).

Bradshaw's book includes a powerful meditation technique that involves seeing the house you lived in as a child and then inviting the child to talk to you. An adaptation of this exercise is included in today's assignment.

Assignment

Before working with your Inner Child, you need to find or develop the Nurturing Parent or Healthy Adult part of yourself. That part is an emotionally mature adult, has compassion, and is connected to Spirit; it can be your Higher Self.

Begin by listing ten good things about yourself. If your Loving Presence/God/Higher Power were to list ten positive characteristics about you, what might those be? Write them down. If *compassionate* or *loving* or *supportive* are not on your list, can you find that part of you that is compassionate, loving, or supportive? Think of a time you displayed these traits, and feel them within yourself now. Know these qualities belong to you—at least some of the time—add them to your list.

Read through your ten positive characteristics and affirm each one for yourself. For example, if you wrote *honest* as one of your qualities, say aloud, *I am honest.* Make sure at least one thing you say is *I am compassionate*, or *I am loving*, or *I am supportive.*

Great. Now declare every asset out loud again, but this time slow it down, take a breath after each one so you can take in the vibration of the words and allow them to really sink into your consciousness. As you say and own these words, you are building and strengthening your

Healthy Adult self, which must be present before going on to the next exercise.

◆

This second exercise uses guided imagery, and through it you'll go back to your childhood home and see the young child who was you. You might want to audiotape the directions or have someone else read them so you can experience this as a closed-eye exercise.

Get comfortable, with your spine straight, and focus on your breath for a few moments. In your mind's eye, picture the earliest home that you can remember—where you grew up or spent at least a part of your early childhood.

Still using your imagination, look at the house from the outside—the lawn, the backyard, perhaps a swing set or sandbox. Bring in as much detail as you can remember. Is the house constructed of brick or aluminum siding, wood or stone? If there are flowers, imagine smelling them now. If you walked barefoot on the grass, feel it under your feet now. If there was a swing on the porch, feel yourself swinging. What other details do you remember?

Imagine going to the front door, opening it, and entering the house. See the layout—where is the front room or living room? The kitchen? The bedrooms? See the furniture of your childhood, the linoleum or carpeting or hardwood floors, the wallpaper or paint, the drapes or blinds. Go from room to room. Where did you watch TV? See that room now. Visually explore the kitchen or dining room, wherever you ate your meals. Look at your bedroom and see your prized objects: A teddy bear? A pennant on the wall? Your favorite doll? A special toy? See your clothes in the closet and drawers. Take some time to look all around the house—include the basement and attic if you had either.

Hear the sounds of the house: the wind whistling through the trees, the chirping of the birds, the voices of your family members. Is there singing? Shouting? Both? Or maybe there is a disconnected silence?

Where would you be in that house? Find yourself, the younger you. What is the child doing? Feeling? Saying? Are Mom and Dad there, too? Siblings? Other relatives? Just observe the child for a little while.

When you are ready, see yourself as you are now—in the role of the Healthy Adult—and enter the picture. Tell the youngster that you are the adult from the child's future. Explain to this Inner Child that you are the Nurturing Parent and have come to take care of the child.

When you and the child are ready, take the youngster's hand and lead the child away from the other people in the house. See you, the Nurturing Adult, and the young child walk out of the house, hand in hand. Through the front door, down the walk, and onto the sidewalk.

Bring this youngster back to where you are right now. Holding the child on your lap, take a few minutes to express love, affection, and caring.

Next, imagine this child getting smaller and smaller, becoming so tiny you can hold the child in the palm of your hand. Then gently place the child into your heart.

Take a deep breath. Smile as you glance down at your chest. Your Inner Child is now in your heart, where the youngster can feel nurtured, protected, and cherished.

After doing this guided imagery exercise, you now have a tiny being dependent on you, a little one who lives in your heart. Be protective of this Inner Child. With your hands on your heart, talk to the child and listen to the responses. If you have a photo of yourself as a youngster, look at it as you connect with your Child Within. This can be powerful and transformative, and it might take courage to stay with all the feelings of the Inner Child.

Every day make it a point to touch in with this little one within you. You can do this with a simple "Hi, sweetie" or with a longer conversation. The next section teaches a new communication skill to use with your Child Within.

Day (14) Right-Hand/Left-Hand Dialogue

One of my favorite tools to connect to my Inner Child is Right-Hand/Left-Hand Dialogue, a technique described in Lucia Capacchione's *Recovery of Your Inner Child*. Although it feels awkward, write questions with your dominant hand (DH), the hand you usually write with, and answer them with your nondominant hand (NH). The DH is linked to the left side of the brain—the logical, rational part. The NH is linked to the more creative, more intuitive right side of the brain. As you switch your pen or pencil back and forth between hands, you link your conscious knowing to your subconscious understanding. The Healthy Adult hand (DH) can ask questions and then get answers from a subconscious part, the Inner Child, who is using the NH. It allows words to surface that the conscious mind might never have had a clue about.

Our words and actions begin at an unconscious level. Freud and other psychologists have theorized that only 10 percent of what we do comes from a conscious place. Just like the iceberg—there is a small amount sticking out (conscious) and a large amount (unconscious) beneath the surface. Is it any wonder, then, that when your conscious voice says something like *I am going to choose healthy foods and lose weight,* there might be a lot beneath the surface negating your intention?

Whenever I teach the Right-Hand/Left-Hand Dialogue technique to my clients, I make sure they understand that the adult (the DH) must come from a place of nonjudgment and love. In order for the other parts to open up and be truthful, this adult part—the Nurturing Parent part that you worked on in the first part of the previous assignment—needs to be compassionate and understanding.

Read through this whole section before attempting to use this for yourself.

With your DH, take your pen or pencil and write a question to the young child you once were—your Inner Child. Then immediately switch your pen or pencil to the other hand, your NH. Write whatever comes to you without censoring it. The action will feel awkward and the words will probably look like scribble-scrabble, and that's fine. Just do it without thinking about it. When that hand feels done, switch to your DH to respond. Continue back and forth, ending with the adult, the DH, thanking the Inner Child for communicating with you.

My first experience with Right-Hand/Left-Hand Dialogue allowed me to connect at a very deep level to my Child Within. I was delighted she was not only willing to converse with me but also trusting enough to tell me what she was feeling and needing. Our conversation went something like this:

> DH (Dominant Hand): Dear Little Meryl—will you be willing to talk to me?
> NH (Nondominant hand): Yes
> DH: Thanks. I'd like to get to know you better. You are a part of me, and I want to understand and love you.
> NH: Good
> DH: I was wondering—why do you eat so much?
> NH: Because I feel so empty inside.
> DH: What makes you feel good?
> NH: Daddy

I loved my daddy. Although he was strict at times, I knew I was loved and that I was his little girl. When he started to travel for business, it felt like a part of me died or went numb. Before doing this Right-Hand/Left-Hand Dialogue I had not realized that I had felt empty inside as a child and had turned to food to fill the huge cavern. This was very new information for me.

As you continue with the Right-Hand/Left-Hand writing, remember, do not shame the responses you get from the NH, your Inner Child. Instead, always be affirming and loving. The dialogue went on like this:

> DH: Oh, you must have really missed your daddy.
> NH: Yes
> DH [giving the young part empathy]: It is so hard for a little girl to not have her daddy around. I am sorry you felt so alone. Thank you for telling me. I am the

adult who loves you and is always with you. Is there anything I can do for you now?

NH: I want a hug

DH: Sure.

With that, I put down my pen, hugged myself, and dissolved into convulsive sobs. I stayed engulfed in the feelings and even said aloud, "I love you, I love you," over and over again with my arms tightly embracing myself. As I got in touch with my little-girl self, I also felt the depths of her pain—and so began the healing.

Because you can touch into intense, raw feelings in this exercise, you might choose to do it with a mental health professional. If you are going to do it on your own, make sure you are feeling strong and grounded before you start. If you experience severe emotional pain, use one of the tapping techniques to lessen the intensity—stop the writing and go immediately into the EFT setup phrase—"Even though I am feeling _____ [angry, sad, guilty, scared, etc.], I deeply and completely accept myself"—as you tap on the Karate Chop Point.

When your Inner Child identifies a painful memory, your body goes back into the fight-or-flight response. The good news is, once you are conscious of the event and the feelings around it, you can neutralize it. Dr. David Feinstein, a clinical psychologist and national director of the Energy Medicine Institute, explains how tapping heals trauma in his DVD *Introduction to Energy Psychology*:

> Bringing to mind a traumatic memory renders the receptor that maintains the fear pathways vulnerable to disruption. (You can only change

what you've activated. Something happens when you activate the memory that makes it vulnerable to being erased.) Tapping the acupressure points (also called acupoints) sends signals that eradicate those receptors.

Furthermore, Dr. Dawson Church (mentioned in chapter 5) maintains that the tapping interrupts the conditioned response loop and tells your brain that you are safe.

Occasionally, just tapping the Karate Chop Point will be enough. If not, go through the whole EFT protocol or use the RITT script. If you want, you can imagine tapping on the young-child part of yourself. Once the feelings have subsided, resume the Right-Hand/Left-Hand Dialogue.

My first experience with Right-Hand/Left-Hand Dialogue spurred me to connect with my Inner Child on a daily basis. The more I took on the role of a Nurturing Parent—avoiding criticism and judgment and instead being praiseful, loving, soft, and compassionate—the more my Inner Child revealed to me what troubled her and what she wanted and needed.

I discovered that my Inner Child, Little Meryl, was often afraid and had learned to put on a happy face and not tell anyone about her fears. I found out that she didn't know how to relate to others very well—she knew how to give them what they wanted, but she had no idea how to be herself and stay in her own truth. During this time of discovering my forever-young self, Cabbage Patch dolls were the rage, and I purchased one to symbolize Little Meryl. Although it might seem strange to some, when I was home alone I carried her around and talked to her in loving terms. Whenever I did the Right-Hand/Left-Hand Dialogue exercise, I placed the doll in a chair facing me. You might also want to find a physical representation of your Inner Child or a photo of your younger self.

Assignment

It's time for you to try out the Right-Hand/Left-Hand Dialogue for yourself. What information would you like from a younger part or a subconscious part? Remember, the DH is your Nurturing Adult part, and your NH can access the unconscious or subconscious, your Inner Child part. If the NH releases big feelings that are hard to deal with, use EFT or RITT to reduce the emotional charge.

A good starting line is this, to be written by the DH: *Hi, _____ . Will you be willing to talk to me today?* Switch hands and allow your NH to write whatever flows, whatever it wants to write, without conscious thought and without editing. You can also draw pictures, doodle, whatever that young part wants to do to get comfortable communicating with the adult you in this way. Put the pen in your DH, and respond with praise and affirmations whenever possible. Keep going—asking who, what, where, when, and why questions with your dominant hand and allowing the nondominant hand to answer them. If the responses are unclear, continue to probe, responding with empathy and understanding. When you feel complete, end with the adult part thanking the child part.

Write to the Inner Child daily—even if it is just a few sentences. You are getting access to subconscious parts of yourself and re-parenting the Child Within.

Day ⑮ Parts Work—Embracing the Inner Critic

Having internal voices doesn't mean we are loony; it just means we have different parts of ourselves. In the counseling field, working with the various aspects is known as ego-state therapy.

You have experienced dealing with the Inner Child and the Nurturing Adult. Now we will focus on the Inner Critic, also known as the Critical Parent. That's the part of you that either quietly demeans you, *You should _____,* or screams contemptuous epithets in your head, *You stupid idiot*—or both. For many of us, the voice has been a constant companion since childhood. We are so used to the continuous clatter and chatter of negative self-talk that we might not even consciously notice it. It's the low-level drone in the background that is always there.

The Inner Critic sees only your faults. If you accomplish 90 percent of your goals, it will holler at you about the other 10 percent. This voice puts you down, blames you when things don't work out right, and is a horrendous taskmaster. Although not everyone in the world has an overly harsh Inner Critic, every compulsive overeater I have ever counseled had a very powerful, influential one.

Why and how would such a voice be a part of most of us? As children grow up, parents want them to do their best and point out ways to improve. As part of "civilizing" their children, mothers and fathers teach them how to behave properly, how to look good, how to best fit into the world. And parents have help in this task—teachers, family members, clergy, and society in general all collude with the parents in the shaping of the children. None of this is done with pernicious intent—it is the means of creating youngsters that the parents and society will be proud of.

In the process, though, children often deduce that they are not okay the way they are—there is something about them that needs to be fixed in order to be acceptable. The fault-finding voice that they hear becomes internalized, and as the children grow they develop an Inner Critic based on what they've heard and the conclusions they've come to. In an attempt to make sure you don't become a pariah, that voice tells the child (and later, the adult) such things as:

- It's not okay to make a mistake.
- If you goof up, people will reject you.
- You are no good at that.
- You will never amount to anything.
- You are selfish and inconsiderate.
- You are stupid.
- You are worthless.
- You don't matter.
- You are fat and ugly.
- No one likes you.

Even though it says such debasing things, the Inner Critic actually came into being in an attempt to aid you—so that your behavior would be respectable and you would be able to fit in and not be ostracized. That part wants to help you avoid pain, shame, and rejection. It wants you to be the most perfect person possible so that others won't criticize you, and it came into being to protect you from hurt and disappointment.

In working with your Inner Critic, you will call on your Healthy Adult part—the part of you that is emotionally mature as well as compassionate and understanding. If you have just eaten a Twinkie, for instance, the Inner Critic might lash into you: "I can't believe you did that. You are such a loser. You are bad. You are pathetic. You are fat and ugly and no one will be your friend."

The Healthy Adult, on the other hand, feeling compassionate and choosing to understand the needs beneath the action, might say, "I know you are feeling really bad about that. You were under a lot of stress and maybe you were feeling hungry, angry, lonely, or tired, all triggers to overeat. Please stop beating yourself up. You really are a child of God, and I love you. I don't want you to be so unhappy with yourself. Let's look at what happened before you ate the Twinkie and figure out why you wolfed it down."

It is important to continue to practice using and hearing the voice of the Healthy Adult. If you have trouble coming up with words of encouragement, think of what you say to your own children, nieces or nephews, or neighborhood kids when you are in a place of love, patience, and compassion.

When the Inner Critic is doing its thing, you can begin to discover the needs beneath the put-downs by separating the Inner Critic voice from that of the Healthy Adult. Similar to the Right-Hand/Left-Hand Dialogue, parts work disentangles the different voices within you. This time, though, the parts vocalize their words rather than writing them. Two of my favorite techniques to use for this are Chair Work and Two Hands Talking.

Chair Work

My client, Jane, had a screaming Inner Critic, and she expressed frustration at her inability to silence it. During our meetings, we explored Jane's concern of not fitting in well with her peers, and she recognized her Inner Critic as her mother's voice—but it was louder and more insistent than any words that her mom had actually uttered. Jane's Inner Critic badgered her constantly, pointing out and embellishing any defects or blemishes.

Jane agreed to work with her different parts, and we opted to try Chair Work first. Using one chair to represent her Inner Critic and the other chair to assume the role of her Healthy Adult, Jane drew something to represent each voice. For the Inner Critic, she drew a big black X; to represent the Healthy Adult, she wrote, "I love you." The coaching I did with her before we began helped her separate out the voices, so that she could hear the Inner Critic and know that it wasn't her true Self. Jane began by sitting in the Inner Critic chair, and she started a dialogue. As the parts dialogued with each other, Jane moved back and forth from one chair to the other:

> Inner Critic (IC): Aren't you the hefty one! Look at how your belly protrudes over your pants. You are a real muffin top. I thought you wanted to lose weight. You are as big as a cow. Moo. Moo.
>
> *[Jane was seated in the IC chair as she shouted this, in a nasty tone, to the Healthy Adult chair. Then she*

switched chairs, to speak from the Healthy Adult's voice.]

Healthy Adult (HA): Why are you always picking on me? Every time I look in the mirror, all I hear are your criticisms. It sounds like you want me to have a perfect figure. Why is that important to you?

IC [loud voice]: You keep gaining weight, and soon your clothes won't fit. You will hate yourself then. Look at the size of your thighs, Miss Thunder Thighs. You are a fat slob. How could you let yourself go like that? Shame on you! No one will want to be with you.

HA: Why do you think others won't want to be with me if I have an extra bulge or two?

IC: They will reject you and make fun of you when you have fat hanging out, Miss Moo-Moo.

HA: So, you are concerned with my being liked, and my not being hurt by others?

IC: Yes. You are fat and ugly.

HA: I have lots of friends who also have the so-called muffin top. Do you see them as not fitting in or as being inadequate?

IC: No, but I am concerned for you. I don't want anyone to make fun of you behind your back.

HA: Thank you for your concern. The only one making fun of me is you. I think you are here to help and protect me, but you are really horrible to me. I don't like it at all. I wonder if you could do it differently.

IC: What does that mean?

HA: You blast me about the extra weight I am carrying and it doesn't help! I want to find a way to love myself just the way I am . . . Maybe I can put my hands on my belly and send it love. Yes, that's a good idea! When I hear your criticism, I need to remind myself that it is the Inner Critic speaking and not my true Self.

IC: But I want you to look good so others will accept you.

HA: Others do accept me. My goal now is for me to accept me. Although I know you mean well, your voice is brutal. Your intention might be good, but I need to love myself just the way I am regardless of what you say.

IC: I only want to help you.

HA: I appreciate your wanting to keep me safe from hurt. I just don't want to feel so criticized anymore. I am going to try hearing you differently.

IC: What do you mean?

HA: When I hear your voice, I want it to remind me to love myself.

IC: WHAAAT?

HA: You are quick to point out the defects. I would like each real and imagined fault that you bash me with to now remind me that I am

perfectly imperfect. So when you do your thing—
trumpeting my flaws—my goal is to remember it
comes from a place of caring. Even though it may
be your job, please, just say it once. Don't belabor
it, and don't be so mean. Will you agree to that?

IC: I don't know . . . We'll see.

HA: Thank you for talking to me. Now it is up to
me to hear you differently.

After doing this exercise, Jane voiced her appreciation for
being able to recognize the Inner Critic and dialogue with it
rather than just trying to ignore it or banish it. Within a few
weeks, Jane recounted that now when she heard the Inner
Critic start up, she would identify the voice and then smile,
lighten up, and say to herself, "Oh, it's my Inner Critic—
doing its job again!" She was delighted that the critical words
no longer sucked her energy; instead, she used that caustic
voice as a prompting to send love to her body.

Two Hands Talking

Similar to the Chair Work discussed above, another option
is to use your hands to represent the two inner voices. Allow
one hand to speak for the Inner Critic (IC) and the other
hand to be the Healthy Adult (HA). Instead of going back
and forth between two chairs, you stay still and have each
hand "speak" to the other, holding the hand up and moving
the fingers as if it were a puppet speaking. Some of my clients prefer this method, and you will have the opportunity
to try it for yourself to see which one you like better.

Assignment

Start to become more fully aware of the Inner Critic's voice. It is imperative to separate out that voice, knowing that it is not the real Self. Answering the following questions can help (example answers are given in italics):

1. When do you criticize yourself or beat yourself up?
   When I make a mistake.

2. What words does the Inner Critic use at those times?
   You are stupid or dumb. Sometimes it's in the first person: *I am so stupid or I am so dumb.*

3. Who used to say the same type of words to you?
   I don't remember ever being called dumb or stupid. But I had that feeling when I made a mistake—the way my parents would look at me or scold me, without the actual name-calling.

4. If a Loving Presence were to say something to you when you made a mistake, what might that be?
   Oh well, you'll do better next time. It's not that big a deal.

Read through your responses and begin to get an ear for the voice of the Inner Critic, knowing that although it wants to protect you, it has overstepped its bounds. And then, to understand it better, continue on to the next exercise.

◆

Before you begin your Chair Work, set two chairs facing each other. On each chair, place or draw a symbol to represent the voice "sitting" on that chair. For example, the Inner Critic's symbol could be a hammer (a real hammer or a pictorial representation of one) or a whip, and the Healthy Adult's symbol might be a picture of a heart or a smiling sun. (Note: You could give the second chair to your Higher Power instead, and your self-compassionate words will be as if Spirit were talking.)

Have a seat in the Inner Critic's chair, and start a dialogue with the Healthy Adult. Begin giving voice to your judgments—about your weight, what you ate, work, money, children, spouse, family members, friends, acquaintances, colleagues, whatever you are disapproving of right now. In a critical voice, talk to the other chair in the second person, like this: "You are _____ ."

Switch to the Healthy Adult/Spirit chair, and reply to the Inner Critic. Look at the first chair and remember the words that flowed out in acidic tones—the judgments, the blame, and the loathsome feelings. In your most compassionate voice, please talk to the person in the first chair, attempting to use words filled with love and acceptance. Try to discover the needs beneath the contempt that was just expressed.

Go back to the Inner Critic chair, and continue the conversation. Allow those words of understanding and compassion to flow into you. How do you feel? What do you want to say? You might still have more to get off your chest. Say it now. Don't hold anything back.

Switch chairs a fourth time, and in the loving voice of the understanding Healthy Adult, respond to the words you just heard.

Continue moving back and forth between the two chairs until you have expressed all your feelings, from both sides, and have taken in the words of understanding. Allow the Healthy Adult to have the last word, so that it expresses gratitude for the Inner Critic's communicating.

Consider what you have learned about the Inner Critic. Were you able to come to an agreement? Has it changed the way you hear its words?

◆

Finding another issue or expanding on the Chair Work one, give the Two Hands Talking method a try. One hand will be your Inner Critic and the other your Healthy Adult. Have the two hands face each other and dialogue with each other. As each voice is expressed, move your fingers so that your hands resemble puppets. Upon completion, think about the dialogue. Again, has it changed the Inner Critic or the way you respond to it?

You now have three methods to facilitate a dialogue with your Inner Critic: Right-Hand/Left-Hand Dialogue, Chair Work, and Two Hands Talking. Use these any time you become aware that you are beating yourself up, which means the Inner Critic is doing its job. The Healthy Adult is like a detective, searching for the needs that underlie the criticism. The Inner Critic can then be understood, subdued, or given a new assignment.

Chapter 7

Personal Housecleaning
· ··

Each had his past shut in him like the leaves of a book
known to him by heart; and his friends
could only read the title.
—Virginia Woolf, *Jacob's Room*

OUR PAST IS NOT JUST the past, over and done with. Yester-year continues to weigh on the present, and it can drag you down. In the previous chapter, you went digging for unconscious parts (such as the Inner Child and Inner Critic) from your history so you could work with those aspects. In this chapter you will again be examining the past. This time, though, the focus is on behaviors and actions about which you feel guilt or shame.

As human beings, none of us is flawless. We're not supposed to be. We make mistakes, and when we learn from them, we grow. Sometimes we have glaring faults and imperfections. Sometimes we have minuscule character defects that still cause us and others pain or harm. Within the next several pages, you will be given the chance to examine your shortcomings, admit your offenses, and make amends to those you have hurt. It is a considerable undertaking. It is about stopping the rationalizations, the excuses, and the blaming of others. It is about growing up and being accountable. As you do so, you can purge the guilt and shame you have been carrying maybe for years. You have the opportunity for "getting to know you, getting to know all about you," as they sing in *The King and I*. And, in getting to know and understand yourself better, you'll have a new awareness of your needs and what drives your behaviors. This is significant work in your ongoing process of ameliorating the food obsession.

In chapter 3 we discussed the importance of having a support system, and one of the options I suggested was joining OA, FAA, or another one of the Twelve-Step support groups. My recovery began in those fellowships, where I heard and took to heart, "We are as sick as our secrets." I had lots and lots of secrets—those dark aspects of myself I wanted to keep hidden. I took an enormous leap and began to reveal a few of my secrets to Twelve-Step folks. The rejection I feared didn't materialize. This gave me permission to confess more and more of myself, to allow others (and myself!) to experience my imperfections. And, in so doing, I tiptoed out of the Land of Being Fake (where I had lived for decades) and touched into the Land of Being Real. I often share with my clients Margery

Williams's discussion of being real, from *The Velveteen Rabbit*, because it really resonates with me:

> "What is REAL?" asked the Rabbit one day, when they were lying side by side near the nursery fender, before Nana came to tidy the room. "Does it mean having things that buzz inside you and a stick-out handle?"
>
> "Real isn't how you are made," said the Skin Horse. "It's a thing that happens to you. When a child loves you for a long, long time, not just to play with, but REALLY loves you, then you become Real."
>
> "Does it hurt?" asked the Rabbit.
>
> "Sometimes," said the Skin Horse, for he was always truthful.
>
> "When you are Real, you don't mind being hurt."
>
> "Does it happen all at once, like being wound up," he asked, "or bit by bit?"
>
> "It doesn't happen all at once," said the Skin Horse. "You become. It takes a long time. That's why it doesn't happen often to people who break easily, or have sharp edges, or who have to be carefully kept. Generally, by the time you are Real, most of your hair has been loved off, and your eyes drop out and you get loose in the joints and very shabby. But these things don't matter at

all, because once you are Real, you can't be ugly, except to people who don't understand."

As I worked the Twelve Steps, I let go of the bogus me and explored my realness. I found that as I peeled off layers of deceit and became more self-honest, others embraced the authentic me.

It is beyond the scope of this book to discuss all Twelve Steps here. However, the content and assignments presented in this chapter are adapted from three of the Steps and will guide you into dropping self-deception and becoming more real, too.

Day (16) Mini Inventory

Who you are today is a sum total of your previous experiences. Some of those experiences you would like to broadcast from the rooftops with pride. Other experiences, however, you may be ashamed of and wish you could continue burying in the sand. It is time to own all your behaviors, no matter what you did or how awful you think they are. This is the time to examine your past—looking at who you've been and what you've said or done—and hone in on those things you feel guilty or remorseful about. The purpose is not to keep you ensnared in the pit of shame, but to free you from it by beginning to appreciate yourself and to have compassion for what you did and who you were at that time.

Members of Twelve-Step groups are encouraged to write a personal Fourth-Step moral inventory discussing ways they have harmed others and themselves. *The Big Book* explains:

> Next we launched out on a course of vigorous action, the first step of which is a personal house-cleaning, which many of us had never attempted. Though our decision [for us, deciding to stop the emotional overeating] was a vital and crucial step, it could have little permanent effect unless at once followed by a strenuous effort to face, and to be rid of, the things in ourselves which had been blocking us. Our liquor [emotional eating] was but a symptom. So we had to get down to causes and conditions (63–64).

This is true confessions time. It is sobering to take a look at our personality defects, or what I like to call our character traits that have outlived their usefulness. It is very common to blame another for our behaviors or to become defensive, and it is very challenging to take personal responsibility. Doing so, however, helps to strengthen our spiritual muscle and is surely a sign of emotional growth and maturity.

When I was a struggling member of a Twelve-Step fellowship, I knew I had to write a Fourth-Step inventory and come clean about my little bads as well as my judgmental thinking and shameful behaviors. AA says resentment is the number one reason individuals relapse. Therefore, I started with that: I thought about all the people and things I resented, and the length of the list astounded me. Memories popped up from childhood: I resented having to schlep my tagalong sister with me when I played with my friends; I resented having to go to Sunday School; I resented my mother dressing my sister and me in identical clothes; I resented my parents for putting me on diet after diet; I resented having to babysit my siblings; and I certainly resented that my brother didn't listen to me when I babysat. As I wrote, I was surprised at the number of resentments I had been carrying. I hadn't told anyone about these—I hadn't even admitted them to myself.

I chose other character liabilities to write about, too. For instance, I admitted to myself that I liked to be in charge and that my controlling behavior often strained my relationships with others. I scanned through my memory bank, noting specific times that this played out. Even when I was a child, friends complained that I was too bossy.

Then I decided to look at the Seven Deadly Sins and realized, to my horror, that I had exemplified each one! At first, some seemed foreign—like when I looked at the word *envy* and attempted to convince myself that I was never envious and this trait didn't apply to me. In spite of this, I picked up the pen and I wrote, "Envy. This isn't something that rings true for me. How have I been envious? Who have I been envious of?" Forcing myself to write about this, I discovered that I had felt envious as a child, such as when my brother was born. He was the big deal, and, to my young mind, his sisters were nothing in comparison. Although I had thought envy didn't apply to me, once I got started, I found myself writing and writing about it, releasing pent-up feelings.

Stop Eating Your Heart Out

I have heard it said, "The deception of others is nearly always rooted in the deception of self." Becoming conscious of each character defect was extremely hard for me—a young woman who had prided herself on being as flawless as possible. What a mask I wore, and it was so molded to me that I often lost track of the real versus the artificial me.

Delving into more personality flaws, I realized my outward holier-than-thou attitude was camouflaging my real feelings of inadequacy and worthlessness. I was able to examine the shadow parts of myself, the less-than-pretty parts that I had closed my eyes to. I chose to open my eyes and face those darker, not very nice, aspects. Writing about past behaviors (that I had furtively wished could stay hidden forever) allowed me to begin to decipher myself better—my motivations, my concerns, my wants, and my needs.

Completing this exercise was one of the most difficult things I have ever pushed myself to do. It took a lot of self-discipline and resolution. It was hard to admit that I had personality defects and then surprising to see all the poisonous words spew forth on my paper. I was finally able to acknowledge my less-than-perfect behaviors and my less-than-perfect self. I am so glad I took the plunge—it was a cathartic experience, to come clean to myself and own that I had these negative characteristics. I applauded myself that I had the courage to do it, and I also felt somehow lighter and freer as a result of putting the words on paper.

Assignment

Although I wrote a full moral inventory as suggested in AA, my clients (and you) are instructed to write only a mini inventory. Now it's your turn to dig into your past and reveal yourself to you. A person often carries shame and feels defective based on unresolved guilt, and it is about time to acknowledge where you "sinned." The original meaning of *sin*, by the way, is simply "to miss the mark." (At the Greek Olympics in archery, when the arrow missed the bull's-eye, someone yelled "sin.")

Let's begin with the so-called Seven Deadly Sins. This is a mini inventory, so you need only list a few examples for each.

Gluttony: This one applies to all of us, doesn't it! Write about a few times when you ate or drank to excess. What were the triggering events and emotions? How did you feel as a result of the gluttonous behavior?

Wrath: Are you holding grudges? Are there people you hope to get even with? What about self-righteous anger? Misdirected anger? Are you impatient with others' faults? Again, choose a few to write about and examine.

Sloth: In what ways have you been spiritually lazy? How have you not made healthy changes in yourself? Write about a few.

Envy: Whom have you envied? Why? What do they have that you covet?

Greed: In what ways have you been greedy in the past? What were the underlying needs? Have you been able to give without having expectations of others? Do you have an underlying desire for power?

Pride: Do you feel you are better than someone? Worse than someone? When has your ego caused some negative ramifications? What feelings were underneath?

Lust: Have you been promiscuous? Have you misused sex or been unfaithful? Were there consequences? What do you suppose was the motivation? Unmet needs? Has a self-destructive drive for pleasure harmed yourself or others?

If any of the words don't seem to resonate, write anyway. As I mentioned earlier, when I saw the word *envy*, I thought I had nothing to say—and then I started writing and surprised myself with all that I unearthed. So even if the word doesn't seem to apply to you, begin writing anyway.

Think of behaviors you are ashamed of. How did you go against your morals or ethics or those of society? What did you do? What was your motivation? Your thoughts and feelings? What character traits were exhibited? This is about getting to know and understand yourself better.

Is there anything else you need to admit to yourself? Are there other areas in which you have been less than the person you want to be? Are there other defects of character? Choose all the flaws you are willing to explore.

Set aside time to work on this. It can be helpful to look at old photos and address books to help jog your memory. For now, what you write is just for your eyes, so keep your writing in a safe and secure place. Don't worry about spelling or punctuation—just write.

Day ⑰ Giving It Away

Congratulations! If you completed the assignment from Day 16, you are to be commended for your honesty, perseverance, and courage. It takes a lot to recall those things that feel shameful. Owning your shadow parts, though, allows you the opportunity to heal those aspects that fill you with remorse.

As challenging as it was for you to write your mini inventory, it will probably be even more difficult for you to let someone else know what you wrote. Yes, it is time now, once you get to today's assignment to give it away. You might be thinking that writing it was enough and you don't need to go further. Discussing what you've written with another person, however, is paramount for your healing. It allows you to be totally honest with another human being, and that person may provide useful feedback to help you come to terms with your past behaviors.

Begin to think about whom you might entrust with your confidences. If you are active in your church, you can go to your clergy. If you are currently in therapy, you'll probably confide in your therapist. If you have a trustworthy friend who will listen without judgment and without the need to fix you or solve your problems, you might choose that person. Do not select an individual who, upon hearing your disclosures, will be hurt. It needs to be someone who can objectively hear you and, like the Healthy Adult or Nurturing Parent we worked with earlier, be compassionate and understanding.

Before getting together with this other person, first spend some quiet time with your Higher Power, reading what you have written. As you tell this Loving Presence about the mistakes you have made and the personality flaws you have observed, you are also admitting them to yourself. Nothing can be consciously changed unless it is acknowledged, and you are now disclosing to yourself, your Higher Power, and a support person what you did, how you felt about it, and what you've learned. No more rationalizations. No more blaming another. And, as a fringe benefit, as you continue to unravel your motives and figure yourself out, you'll move into a place of greater self-acceptance, which is a precursor to self-love.

When it was time for me to discuss my inventory with another human being, I balked. Let somebody in close? Reveal myself and my darkness? Ouch. I don't think so!

But I wanted to stop my food compulsion, and I believed that coming clean about the real me—including all the parts I wanted to hide—would help. I spent some quiet time talking to my Higher Power and admitting my wrongs. As I read each item aloud, I was also finally acknowledging to myself exactly what I had done. Although I began reading in a critical voice (my Inner Critic was having a ball), my tone changed as I read. It became softer, gentler. Somehow, I unconsciously switched into the Healthy Adult. I recognized the feelings and unmet needs behind each action. I saw the younger version of myself that was admitting her faults, and I felt compassion for her.

But I still needed to discuss this with another human being. I wondered who I could allow to see the dark crevices that I brought to light when writing my inventory. At that time, I didn't have a clergyman or therapist to discuss this with, so I chose a close Twelve-Step friend whom I trusted. I called Judi and told her that I wanted to stop emotional overeating and I needed to share with her some of my past shameful behaviors. She agreed, and we set up a time to meet at her home. I didn't want her to come to my house—I wanted to be able to escape in case it got so intense that I felt I had to flee.

Although my Healthy Adult had understood the motivation for past behaviors, the Inner Critic had once again returned and was doing her thing as I drove to Judi's house: *How can you admit to Judi all the things you've done? You're disgraceful, and she will reject you,*

Judi lovingly welcomed me and intuitively knew I needed to get right down to business. With great trepidation, I sat face-to-face with her, took out the many pages I had written, and began to share. As I read, I glanced up periodically to see if she was giving me looks of condemnation. Instead, I saw only love and understanding. Revealing myself to her was huge for me, and I felt vulnerable and totally naked. When I finished reading, we discussed the motivations, the feelings, and the needs. Judi, thankfully, did not judge me—she was supportive, noncritical, and very kind. The comforting warmth I received through her empathy and compassion blanketed me, and I was able to relax, feeling an immense sense of relief.

Upon completion, she gave me a long, strong, tender hug and then said something that stayed with me: "Yes, you did all those things, and they are part of your past. Congratulations for being so honest and open. Now you are free. The past is now really the past. The guilt and shame had weighted you down, and now, with this big release, I bet you'll also be able to release excess body weight."

When I look back, I know it was easy for me to tell my Higher Power because I believed down to the core of my being that I was loved unconditionally. I didn't have too much of a problem telling myself because as I wrote about each item, I was admitting it to myself, and my Healthy Adult part was very affirming. But telling another person was a big, heart-stopping deal—yet I lived through it!

Many of my clients are involved in a Twelve-Step Program, and I have heard numerous Fourth-Step inventories over the years. One client, Stella, sobbed and sobbed as she admitted her anger toward her children in her inventory. Although her troubles occurred more than twenty years ago, Stella vividly remembered countless incidents when her kids' behaviors "got to her," and she wanted to bash her children against the wall. She said it happened over and over, and she was terrified that she was capable of such violence. Although Stella had murderous thoughts, they remained thoughts, not actions. Even though thoughts have energy, I needed to assure Stella that all parents lose their cool from time to time, some to the point of feeling like they are ready to abuse their children. I consoled the still-crying Stella that these were thoughts and not deeds. My words seemed to penetrate, and her weeping ended and her posture changed. Stella began to accept that she had been a frustrated young mother and that, although she had thoughts of hurting her children, she did not act on them. As she walked out of my office, it was obvious that a weight had been lifted from her shoulders.

Celia also noticed a great difference after she discussed her mini inventory with me. She admitted that she had been very greedy in life—always taking the largest serving of food for herself and hiding food from her family. As she talked about several instances, she was filled with remorse and said she hated that she did this. When we probed what might be behind these actions, Celia explained that her older brother was a bully, and throughout their childhood, he grabbed Celia's food or treats for himself. Her parents scolded her brother, but his behavior continued. At a very young age, Celia made a decision that as an adult she would always come first, be served first, and get the biggest portion. Looking at the roots of her "greedy" behavior gave Celia compassion for herself and the motivation to do Inner Child work with her young, fearful part. Although we had worked on food issues for a while, Celia credits the inventory work as being the major breakthrough in her food addiction.

Assignment

Read your inventory to your Higher Power, making sure it is a Loving Presence. Take on the ears of the Healthy Adult as you hear the words being read. Are you able to find some compassion and empathy for your past actions?

Consider who would be an uncritical person with whom you can share all the shortcomings you wrote down. It could be a priest, a counselor, or a trusted friend. Pick somebody who will be tolerant and not condemning. Make sure that the individual is someone who will not be harmed by hearing your inventory.

Take a breath. Yes, now. Sit and breathe. I know how scary it can be to admit to anyone the truth of who you are and what you have done wrong.

When you meet with this person, read and discuss what you have written.

When you are finished, give yourself a huge pat on the back for your honesty and courage, and maybe find a non-food reward for yourself (go to the movies, buy yourself a little something, get a pedicure or massage, etc.).

Day 18 Making Amends

Many emotional overeaters have trouble effectively relating to others and may be deficient in relationship-building skills. For a long time, I recognized that my social skills were stunted, but I thought it was just me. As a counselor, though, I have become very aware that my emotional overeater clients often have relationship problems, too. When our time is spent obsessing over food or eating compulsively, we often choose to isolate. And, since our primary relationship is with food, our personal relationships suffer.

Today we are going to consider current and past relationships in order to bring to light any patterns that have hurt us or others. Then you will be encouraged to make amends, which means not just saying "I'm sorry," but also making changes in your behavior.

When you wrote your mini inventory on Day 16, you identified situations in which you were at fault and the people you had harmed. In today's assignment, you'll acknowledge the hurt you caused, take action to rectify the damages or repay the losses, and then adjust your future actions accordingly.

As I followed the Twelve-Step Program, I was urged to work each step completely. The notion of making amends, however, threw me into a dither. I thought there was no way I could make amends—that would mean I'd have to admit to the individual that I was wrong or had damaged them. Since I had spent my life trying to be right all the time and look good, this was a seemingly impossible task. Fear, shame, and guilt washed over me just thinking about it. I had written my inventory, but this step had me admitting I was wrong to the person involved, and I didn't think I could muster the courage to do it.

Since I wanted to end my food obsession, however, I decided to take the first action and just make a list of the people I had injured. I dutifully went through my inventory and gathered names, and I also endeavored to remember all whom I had hurt by my words and deeds even outside those I'd inventoried, and added them to my list. The next part, though, seemed impossible—to contact these people and make direct amends to them. Oh my goodness, how could I do that?

Taking a deep breath, I thought maybe I'd be able to start with one of the easy ones: As a teen, I shoplifted a bagel cutter from the local department store. To make amends, I sent a dollar bill (the cost of the item) in the mail, with an explanatory note. That was simple and caused no fear. If only all the amends could be this easy, I mused.

The thought of contacting people I knew and making amends to them filled me with dread. I spent time in prayer and meditation seeking the courage to proceed. As the fear level dropped a smidge, I got bolder and considered what I might be willing to do next. Many of my amends had to do with food I stole, mainly for binges.

I put my parents on the top of the list. When they went out of town, I (as an adult) checked their house every few days to make sure everything was in order. They asked me and I was happy to oblige—eager, even. Because whenever I went to their empty house, by myself, I searched through every cupboard seeking "good" (binge) foods and helped myself to them. I would open the freezer and, by george, those pastries seemed to jump right into my hand and then down my gullet. Many times I stood with the freezer door open, shoving those frigid desserts into my mouth. The texture was cardboard—and the flavor was, too—yet I continued to cram down a ton of frozen baked goods without chewing and without tasting.

Now the time had come for me to make amends to my parents for all the food I had taken without their knowledge. Facing my mother in person was way too scary for me, so I decided to call her to make the amends. Afraid I'd be tongue-tied, I wrote out a little script:

Mom.

Whenever you went out of town, you asked me to watch your house. I used to come over and help myself to food in your cupboards and in your freezer. I ate a lot of the frozen pastry. I am sorry I took it without asking and without telling you. I want to be free of my food compulsion, so I am admitting this and making amends. I am sorry I did this. It won't happen again. Will you forgive me?

Once I had her on the line, I read my mother the script and then stopped breathing, awaiting her response. I thought she'd yell or make a disparaging remark about my weight. Instead she seemed unconcerned and casually replied, "Oh, and all this time I thought your father was noshing on it." I told her that I'd reimburse her for the food I had sneakily consumed, but she declined my offer. Although I had seen this as a mountain, in her eyes it was only a molehill. Whew! Two down, lots more to go!

With that kind of response, I was ready to tackle more amends, and I called my brother and apologized for the ice-cube-tray incident, when I had suggested he put his lip on the tray and his skin stuck to the metal. I also apologized for the bee incident, when a bee landed on my towel and I urged my brother to bring me the towel and he got stung. My brother hardly remembered the occurrences, and he was gracious in accepting my apologies.

I recognized that I was a controller and that I often had a holier-than-thou attitude. For instance, when I heard a member sharing at a Twelve-Step meeting that her favorite binge food was plain M&Ms, I smugly thought, what a waste of calories! After the meeting, I boasted to my friends that I would never stoop so low as to eat plain M&Ms— I only ate the peanut ones so there would be nutritional value. I thought I was better than the speaker because I chose a healthier binge food!

As I made amends, I not only apologized to my friends for having a self-righteous attitude, but I also confessed what was really going on—I had been feeling inferior, so I acted superior; it was all an act. It was very hard for me to own that in myself, and it was very humbling for me to share it with others. I also said that my intent was to change and stop being self-righteous and I'd appreciate their letting me know if they saw me doing it again. Thankfully, my friends accepted my amends and forgave me. This admission paved the way for more genuine relationships.

My clients often recount their experiences of making amends. Every single one of them admitted to being very afraid, and most were very pleased with the results. Gini, for instance, used to lie to her husband almost every time he wanted sex—she'd say she had a headache, her period, she was too tired, etc. She said she loved her husband and wanted to improve their relationship and chose to come clean with her past lies and make amends. Bringing up the subject and confessing her untruths, Gini made amends, and her husband encouraged her to talk about what was causing this behavior. Gini said that they talked for quite some time about her needs and her wants. He not only forgave her but also looked for ways to please her so she'd be more interested in having sex with him.

Ralph made amends to his children for eating all their goodies. The children would bring sweets home from parties and Halloween, and Ralph would confiscate all the treats, telling the kids he only wanted them to eat nutritious foods. Then, in secret, Ralph consumed all the forbidden junk. Now in their twenties, his kids just shook their heads and rolled their eyes when they heard the confession, and they easily forgave their father.

Not everyone you might approach will be as magnanimous. It is our task to make the amends without worrying about the other's response. Rita made amends for having what her mother described as "a big mouth." As a teen, Rita showed disrespect and talked back to her mother and now, as an adult, she chose to make amends for that past behavior. Rita's mother heard the apology and angrily retorted, "Yes, you were a real brat. And you are not much better now." Although her mother was not about to forgive her, Rita did what she needed to do for herself.

Assignment

It is time to write a list of the individuals you have harmed throughout your life, specifying what you did. Don't think about what you are going to do with the list as you write it—just get those names on paper. Have you participated in activities that were in some way hurtful to others? What other people have you injured? Write them on your list. Again, use old diaries, photos, or whatever is useful to bring up recollections from the past. Look back at your inventory from Day 16 and make sure those names are included here, too.

◆

Now that you have written the names, it is time to actually make amends. Scrutinize your list: Would anyone be hurt to hear about what you did? It is not okay to make amends to clear your conscience if the information would be damaging to another. If, for instance, you had an affair, do not go to the other person's spouse and make amends—that would be a case of wounding others.

When you are ready, approach the individual—face to face, by phone, by email, or by snail mail.

- Admit your mistake.
- Ask for forgiveness.
- Take whatever action is appropriate to rectify the wrongdoing.
- Change the behavior.

The person's response is not your concern. Some may be angry; some may be openhearted and forgiving. Whatever the reaction, remember that you are doing this to clear away the wreckage of your past and derail your food obsession.

What if the person you hurt has died? In your meditation, ask to connect to the individual. Or you could go to the person's gravesite and make amends aloud there. Or write a letter to the person and then burn it.

After completing your amends, give yourself a big pat on the back and a big hug. You have just taken a giant step by admitting you harmed someone, remedying the damage done, requesting forgiveness, and changing your behavior. This is not easy stuff and you are doing it, so congratulations to you on your courage. You have worked hard on cleaning up your past wrongs and becoming free of the chains that bound you to them. As you have lifted your guilt and made an attempt at harmony with the other person, you are available to establish better relationships with people from your past as well as with those in the present and those you will meet in the future. And your compulsion to overeat will be diminishing.

When others have injured you, it is important for your own health and well-being to forgive them. We will explore this in the next chapter.

Chapter 8

Conscious Living
. . . .

Not knowing when the dawn will come I open every door.
—EMILY DICKINSON, *"DAWN"*

YOU ARE AMAZING. YOU HAVE completed eighteen days of assignments, with only three days left! It's awesome that you're keeping on keeping on—growing and changing as you work through the assignments. Your relationship with food has been going through a metamorphosis, too. You began this book in the hopes of letting go of your food compulsion, and the journey has been much bigger than that. It has been about opening your eyes to all aspects of yourself—the light as well as the dark—and moving to a place of self-acceptance.

Those who work a Twelve-Step Recovery Program discover that certain Promises start manifesting after they have made their amends. These are enumerated in *The Big Book* and include the following:

- We are going to know a new freedom and a new happiness.
- We will comprehend the word *serenity* and we will know peace.
- Self-seeking will slip away.
- Our whole attitude and outlook on life will change.
- We will intuitively know how to handle situations that used to baffle us.

Although other Promises are also mentioned, you might be most cognizant of these five and delighted in their actualization. Although you have not done all the Steps (unless you are already involved in a Twelve-Step support group), my guess is that you, too, are finding some of the Promises coming true for yourself. If even one of these Promises has come true for you, look how far you have come!

This chapter continues adding elements that support you in living a conscious life: being authentically you. As you have been diligently completing the assignments, your sense of self has undoubtedly been improving. And the more you come to love, accept, and appreciate yourself, the more food will just be food—rather than your drug of choice.

Day (19) Forgiveness

In general, emotional overeaters hold a lot of resentments and grudges. Maybe you remember being snubbed in the third grade or are still incensed about the way so and so treated you. Writing your mini inventory in the last chapter allowed you to clear the majority of old grievances, but I bet there are still people permanently etched in your mind whom you might choose to forgive.

"Resentments rot the container they're in" is a powerful statement that I heard and took to heart years ago. The people we resent might be blissfully living out their lives, with no idea how their actions, inactions, thoughts, or behaviors are eating away at us like a corrosive acid. In the tons of books written on the art and process of forgiveness, the authors all make the same point—forgiveness is for you, not the individual you are forgiving. The internationally renowned speaker Caroline Myss wrote in her best seller *Anatomy of the Spirit*:

> When we harbor negative emotions toward others or toward ourselves, or when we intentionally create pain for others, we poison our own physical and spiritual systems. By far the strongest poison to the human spirit is the inability to forgive oneself or another person. It disables a person's emotional resources. The challenge . . . is to refine our capacity to love others as well as ourselves and to develop the power of forgiveness (84).

Forgiveness is tough. Many of us hold on to our old wounds, hurts, and resentments until they fester and turn us sour and bitter. We refuse to forgive because we have been so wronged. As we remember old hurts, we hope that those who wounded us will eventually wake up and apologize for their grievous behaviors. Too often, we are unmercifully hard on ourselves and need to ease up and forgive our own selves. It's been said that having resentment is like taking poison and waiting for the other person to die. When we refuse to forgive, whom are we really hurting? And can we let go of the bingeing and emotional overeating if we are carrying scads of resentments?

Forgiveness does not mean liking the person who wronged you or condoning the behavior; it means understanding the other person's humanness and releasing the rock of resentment in your heart. Forgiveness is part of self-care—it is an act of freeing one's self. There are a lot of behaviors that seem unforgivable, including rape, incest, murder, and abuse. When atrocities occur, we can choose to hold on to our anger and rage, let them burn a hole inside us, and keep us chained to food and binges. Or we can, at some point, move into the spiritual act of forgiveness.

Several years ago the following story made the rounds on the Internet:

"How Heavy Is Your Bag?"

One of my teachers had each one of us bring a clear plastic bag and a sack of potatoes. For every person we'd refuse to forgive in our life, we were told to choose a potato, write on it the name and date, and put it in the plastic bag. Some of our bags, as you can imagine, were quite heavy. We were then told to carry this bag with us everywhere for one week, putting it beside our bed at night, on the car seat when driving, next to our desk at work.

The hassle of lugging this around with us made it clear what a weight we were carrying spiritually, and how we had to pay attention to it all the time to not forget and leave it in embarrassing places. Naturally, the condition of the potatoes deteriorated to a nasty slime. This was a great metaphor for the price we pay for keeping our pain and heavy negativity. Too often we think of forgiveness as a gift to the other person, and while that's true, it clearly is also a gift for ourselves!

So next time you decide you can't forgive someone, ask yourself, isn't my bag heavy enough?

The Golden Rule admonishes us to "love thy neighbor as thyself." Does that mean we can treat our neighbor as poorly and as harshly as we sometimes treat ourselves? A few days ago, you worked with your Inner Critic, who is good at bashing and blaming you for perceived imperfections. Now it is time, once again, to move into the place of forgiving yourself.

You recently made amends for past behaviors that were immoral, unethical, cruel, or in some way damaging to another, and hopefully the people you contacted have accepted your apologies. But have you forgiven yourself for those past behaviors? Karen Casey, author of the inspirational book *A Life of My Own* reminds us,

> Being human means making mistakes. No doubt we could have been better parents, better lovers,

better employees, surely better children. But we were good enough! Forgiving ourselves for our past transgressions will free us to find more serenity in our present lives. We don't have to let our mistakes, or anyone else's, hold us back any longer (28).

In a meditation a few days ago, I asked myself, "Whom do I need to forgive today?" and the answer was "Myself." *Hmm.* Yes, now I remembered the hostile way I spoke to yours truly the day before. After I critically viewed some digital photos that had just been taken, I thought, *Look at my hair. What a mess! I can't believe I didn't notice it was so flyaway. I should have seen a stylist before having pictures taken.*

And that was just the beginning. The Inner Critic's voice continued: *Oh, my, when I smile broadly there are a ton of wrinkles around my eyes. I look old. I shouldn't smile so much. A small smile would have worked, why did I have to grin? Look at all the wrinkles! Why didn't I try to camouflage them? I should have had a beauty expert over—she would have done my makeup better and made me look good.* Is it any wonder that my usual upbeat mood was gone, and I felt miserable? After all these years, a very strong, very vocal Inner Critic can still show up and drag me down into the darkness of despondency. Once I had awareness of the uproar the critical voice had caused, I decided to move into self-forgiveness. I chose to use the technique of self-empathy and worked with the sad part of myself that believed all the mean words. The dialogue went like this:

Healthy Adult (HA): Boy, you are really upset about the way you look in the new photos.

Sad Part (SP): Yes, I should have seen a stylist and gotten some input from a professional. I hate to look at myself in the new photos.

HA: I know it is very hard for you to accept that you may have made a mistake without beating yourself up.

SP: I should have known better.

HA: Yes, you believe you should have known better. You are disappointed with the way you look in the pictures.

SP: I look fat and old.

HA: So you think you look fat and old. That's your belief. Is it real?

SP: Well . . . I showed a few people the pictures, and they think I look great. Could they be right? I know I am too hard on myself, and my expectations are way too high.

HA: You are hard on yourself, and others commented that you look great in the photos. Is it possible for you to let go of some of your judgment and align with what others have said?

SP: The good news is I trust them, and they are probably right. I am way too much of a perfectionist, and I see my flaws through a magnifying glass. I am glad my friends aren't as judgmental as I am!

HA: Are you able to forgive yourself for your criticalness and being harsh with yourself?

SP: Haha, if I don't, then I'll be beating myself up for being critical. I know how to beat myself up, and I also have made a lot of progress in accepting my imperfections. [sigh] I am just a human being doing the best that I can.

HA: Imagine seeing yourself through your Higher Power's eyes. Is God forgiving or does God hold judgments and criticism about the way you treat yourself?

SP: Oh, that's a good one. When I see myself through God's eyes, I see that I am perfect just the way I am—with all my human foibles.

HA: Great.

SP: I am okay now. I feel good. I'm okay with the photos. Thanks for your help.

HA: You're welcome.

When the Healthy Adult part of me moved into the place of observer, I then gently and lovingly talked to the sad part. Changing my perspective by seeing myself through my Higher Power's eyes immediately shifted my mood.

Holding onto anger and resentments keeps us in victim mode. Though it's not easy, the heroic choice to forgive is an act of self-empowerment and leads to feelings of peace, contentment, compassion, and self-confidence.

Several years ago, my friend and associate Robin Trainor Masci and I attended a Mary Manin Morrissey Dream Builder workshop. Robin and I are both licensed counselors with extensive experience in using energy psychology techniques, and Robin has been a trauma specialist for over thirty years. During one of the workshop segments, Morrissey discussed the importance of forgiveness. Dorothy, the woman next to Robin, stood up and shouted, "There are some things that can never be forgiven. I was gang-raped years ago, and I will never forgive!" Robin suspected there was a reason this woman was seated next to her. During a break, Robin turned to Dorothy and said that she, Robin, was a trauma therapist and asked if Dorothy wanted to clear the emotional charge. Dorothy said she had tried everything and nothing had worked. Robin replied that this might not either, but she asked if Dorothy wanted to give it a try anyway. Dorothy agreed.

They went to a private room to work on it. Dorothy divulged that even though her trauma had happened thirteen years ago, each year her bitterness increased, and it was affecting her marriage and her life. Using the RITT protocol (which Robin and I developed together), Robin asked Dorothy to recount the ordeal, stopping often to tap on acupressure points. After Dorothy concluded, Robin requested that she tell her story again, tapping every time there was *any* emotional discomfort. Dorothy repeated the story several more times, to release any remaining charge. Even though she had to repeatedly tell the details of such a horrific event, Dorothy was thrilled with the results of the tapping and disclosed to Robin that the Higher Power aspect in RITT was of primary importance for her.

Forty-five minutes after Dorothy had left the conference room, she reappeared and walked to the podium at the front of the room. She reminded the attendees of her outburst when she heard that forgiveness was an important spiritual process and then told the group that the energy work she just did took away the charge, asserting, "It's gone!" Although Dorothy acknowledged she wasn't quite ready to forgive, she now saw it as a possibility and could calmly discuss the experience that just a few minutes earlier had caused her to fly into a rage.

A year later, Dorothy contacted us and affirmed that the tapping worked—she could talk about the rape as part of her history, without an emotional charge. And, although she would never condone their behavior, she was now able to forgive her attackers. Dorothy seems to have embodied what Oprah has stated: "Forgiveness is letting go of the hope that the past can be changed."

Hoʻoponopono

In December 2008, Robin and I attended a Hoʻoponopono workshop conducted by Drs. Joe Vitale and Ihaleakala Hew Len. Dr. Hew Len had a strong record of curing the criminally mentally ill using this ancient Hawaiian healing technique. He had accepted a position in the high-security unit at Hawaii State Hospital—which had a very high turnover rate, because the staff feared for its safety while working with these convicted murderers and rapists. Dr. Hew Len agreed to the job as long as the hospital allowed him to work with the patients, the inmates, in his very unique way. He never met face-to-face with them. Instead, as he opened and read their files, he repeated four phrases: "Thank you. I love you. Please forgive me. I'm sorry." Little by little, the patients started getting better.

At the workshop I asked Dr. Hew Len if he was directing those four phrases toward each individual patient, and he clarified that no, he was saying them to himself. As he read the files, feelings would come up in himself—disgust, hate, fear, anger, and so forth. He repeated the four phrases—I love you. I'm sorry. Please forgive me. Thank you.—to clear the feelings within himself. Dr. Hew Len contends that since we are all one, we are responsible not just for ourselves but for anything that comes into our world (including the knowledge of another's misconduct). As we clear ourselves, we evoke the spirit of love and forgiveness. And as we become peaceful, we heal, others heal, and the world around us heals.

Dr. Hew Len calls this process *cleaning*. He told us he is actually saying to himself, "What is going on in me that I am experiencing these problems?" As he went through each of the patient's files, he looked within himself at whatever came up and what he needed to let go of. As he did the cleanings on himself, with no direct patient contact, the patients improved. The inmates' physical shackles and restraints were removed and, within the next few years, the entire ward of criminally insane patients was considered cured, and the ward has been closed. (You can read more about this fascinating story in Vitale and Hew Len's book, *Zero Limits*.)

Ho'oponopono is a forgiveness process in which we take 100 percent responsibility for whatever we experience in our life—with the belief that anything we see or feel comes from within, based on our past memories and the meaning we've made of them. Dr. Hew Len said there is scientific evidence to show that we don't see people as they actually are, but we instead see our own reaction to them. As we do the cleanings, we are asking the Divine to eradicate the memories in our subconscious minds that show up as problems. This process allows us to perceive the world through the eyes of our Creator rather than through the warped eyes of our memories.

During the workshop, when Dr. Vitale was up front presenting, Dr. Hew Len sat in a back corner and disclosed to us that he was cleaning, cleaning, cleaning. He said he does this all day long and recommends that we do it, too, to let go of resentments and achieve a world of peace.

Assignment

If you want to be free of emotional overeating, you cannot afford to hold on to any resentments—not even one!

Make a list of anyone or anything you resent. Go back through the resentments you listed in your mini inventory. Think about your past. Who are you still angry with? Who have you not yet forgiven? In what ways do you need to forgive yourself? Mary Manin Morrissey said, "We all have forgiveness work to do. If you're wondering if this is true, ask yourself, 'Am I breathing?' If the answer is yes, the answer is yes. Ask Spirit, 'Who would you have me forgive today?' Sometimes our hardest forgiveness work is with ourselves." Use the techniques below to get to a place of forgiveness:

- Choose one or both of the tapping techniques (EFT and RITT) to let go of the anger and resentments.

- For self-forgiveness, do parts work, setting a dialogue with your Healthy Adult. Give empathy to the part of you that is angry or sad.

- Selecting one area of discontent, put in practice the Ho'oponopono forgiveness technique, saying over and over again in any order:

"Thank you."

"I love you."

"Please forgive me."

"I am sorry."

Day ⟨20⟩ Gratitude

As a parent, I instructed my children early on to have good manners by saying "please" and "thank you." The words probably didn't mean a whole lot to them at the time, though—they were repeated out of duty—and my kids may not have truly appreciated what they had been given. This makes perfect sense, since I was their role model, and at that time in my life (a young thirty-something), I did not yet embody the quality of gratitude I was trying to instill in them. At that stage in my life, I was selfish and took what I had for granted. This was (obviously) before I had a spiritual awakening.

Upon joining Twelve-Step Recovery, whenever I heard the slogan "Have an attitude of gratitude," I thought I'd puke. I was filled with an emotion that started with a *g* all right, but it wasn't gratitude—it was guilt. Shame, too. My brain told me I had so much to be grateful for, but I was depressed and in despair and could only recognize what I lacked rather than acknowledge my multitude of blessings. To make myself feel even worse, I sashayed right into *shoulding* on myself: *I should feel grateful, I should be happy with what I have, I should not complain, I should appreciate my good fortune.*

As I worked on myself over a period of months and years, my self-image improved, and I was pleasantly surprised to find that I wasn't such a bad person after all. As the shame decreased, feelings of gratitude began to emerge, and I felt thankful for so much—my growth, my health, my family, my recovery, and a bunch more.

The German theologian and mystic Meister Eckhart maintained, "If the only prayer you say in your whole life is 'thank you,' that would suffice." Volumes of books have been written over the centuries extolling the practice of gratitude as a moral rectitude. The latest research, however, shows that being thankful goes way beyond being a spiritual virtue.

Studies have found that being in a state of gratitude benefits our emotional as well as our physical health—it fosters optimism, enhances our immune system, and diminishes the effects of stress. Psychologists Robert Emmons and Michael McCullough conducted a research project (The Psychology of Gratitude, 301-303) on gratitude and thankfulness and ascertained that:

- people who keep weekly gratitude journals exercise more than those who do not keep such journals, feel better about their lives as a whole, have fewer physical symptoms, and are more optimistic;

- those who write gratitude lists make more progress toward their personal goals;

- individuals with neuromuscular disease who do daily gratitude lists have more positive moods, better sleep, and feel more connected to others compared to a control group;

- children who practice grateful thinking are more positive toward their families and school.

After years and years of personal-growth work, I no longer cringe when I hear the word *gratitude*. Just the opposite. Now when I hear or think the word, I become centered and energized. Gratitude is the most important positive feeling I can have—it is a way to thank the Universe for all I have been given. And being grateful clears the way for me to receive even more. Whenever I am feeling troubled or discouraged, if I remember to write a gratitude list, I am able to lift my mood. I just keep writing until I have an attitude shift. You will have a chance to experience this for yourself in today's assignment.

Gratitude elicits an inner smile, reminding me of all the gifts I have received and continue to receive on a daily basis. It takes me outside my little self and allows me to merge with my Higher Self. The Universe is generous and has a lot to give. I am open to receive because I am continually grateful. Now, my reaction to hearing "have an attitude of gratitude" is a far cry from what it used to be.

Reframing

As a counselor, I frequently help my clients do a reframing—seeing the same event through another frame or perspective. It is a lot like the proverbial glass being half-empty or half-full. When life is challenging, that glass may look half-empty (or maybe totally empty!). With that viewpoint, life feels hard and you fall into victim mentality. And when you feel victimized, food starts calling your name again: "I'm here! I'll make you feel better!" is the siren's cry. When you bring gratitude into the equation, you will always see the glass as (at least) half-full. A switch in your perception, a reframe, gives you a more optimistic view of the events in your life, and you will not be pulled back to the food compulsion. As Wayne Dyer says in *Excuses Begone!*, "When you change the way you look at things, the things you look at change." (201)

Yes, stuff happens—tragic events, disappointments, mishaps, and hardships. It is important to get the feelings out right away; it is also important not to dwell in them. There is more than one possible reaction to the happenings in our lives—both those coming from feeling victimized and those rooted in thankfulness. Even if our first reaction is of the poor-me variety, how long does it take to do a reframing and move to a place of gratitude? As we become spiritually more mature, we look for (and often find) the silver lining behind every cloud we encounter. Take a look at the following comments from my clients and me:

> **Event:** The washing machine overflowed.
>
> **Automatic Response:** Oh no! My floor is ruined!
>
> **Reframe:** I am so grateful that now I'll be able to put in the floor I want, and insurance will pay for it!
>
> **Event:** I was in an auto accident.
>
> **Automatic Response:** Oh no! My car is wrecked!
>
> **Reframe:** I am so grateful that I only suffered minor injuries!

Event: My house burned down in a wildfire.

Automatic Response: Oh no! My house has been destroyed.

Reframe: I am so grateful that I only lost material things and that we are safe.

Event: My very young daughter cut her bangs off.

Automatic Response: Oh no! Look what she did to herself—she looks terrible!

Reframe: I am so grateful that she didn't hurt herself with the scissors and that her hair will grow back.

Event: The turkey wasn't cooked in time for the Thanksgiving dinner.

Automatic Response: Oh no! My friends and family are here and ready to eat!

Reframe: I am so grateful that we are not really starving and can make do with all the side dishes and desserts. Or, shall we go out for Chinese food?

Event: I just purchased an expensive plane ticket.

Automatic Response: Oh no! My ticket cost twice as much as I wanted to spend.

Reframe: I am so grateful that I had enough money to purchase the ticket.

Event: I lost my favorite earrings.

Automatic Response: Oh no! I loved those earrings and now they're gone!

Reframe: I am so grateful I got to enjoy those earrings for as long as I did.

You get the idea. Pay attention to the words you use when disappointment or tragedy strikes. At first, most of us are conditioned to react with our *Oh No!* voices, and it's okay to allow those feelings their full strength— for a little bit. After time, though, if we are still feeling victimized, what will help us look for the silver lining?

Challenge yourself to do a reframing, seeking a more desirable interpretation of the event. Change your focus and see it with new, empowered eyes. Staying in the victim mode will be an energy drain and will suck you back into compulsive eating and bingeing over and over again.

Assignment

Use gratitude to help boost your energy. On the 0–10 scale, with 10 being the highest, what is your energy level right now?

Take out a sheet of paper and begin to write things you are grateful for. In this moment, my list would start off like this:

Gratitude List

My senses (sight, taste, hearing, smelling, feeling)

Connection to God

Abundance in my life

My home

My children and grandchildren

My spiritual and biological family

The personal-growth work I've done

My ability to move and walk without pain

Laughter

Music and dance

Write your list and then notice the change in your energy level. Being in a state of gratitude generally gives you an energy boost. Do this exercise whenever you are in a bad mood or notice that your energy level has fallen. And remember, when we are feeling grateful, we aren't reaching for that first compulsive bite.

> Think of a recent or past event about which you still have anger or frustration. Are you able to do a reframing? Can you find the silver lining? Is there anything about that situation for which you are thankful?
>
> Before you go to sleep tonight, think of at least one thing from today that you are grateful for. You can say a little prayer of thanksgiving if you wish.

Day 21 Healthy Eating

You have been diligently working on eliminating your food compulsion, and it is time to take a look at what is okay to eat. Have you ever watched a baby or small child eating? Little children eat until they are full and then stop—they are in tune with their bodies and what they need. As a parent, I vividly remember offering spoonful after spoonful of baby food to my young child. If I pushed in one too many, it came right back out at me!

As we grow up, some of us learn to ignore the signals of being hungry and of being comfortably full. Earlier I mentioned that I lost the ability to feel fullness—my appestat (a part of the human brain thought to regulate hunger), was out of commission. Always rewarded for eating everything on my plate, I focused on my desire to please and squelched my ability to feel full unless I was totally stuffed—and sometimes not even then.

Many books have been written about eating with mindfulness, also called conscious eating or intuitive eating. Dr. Michelle May, author of *Eat What You Love, Love*

What You Eat, discusses eating with intention and attention: Eat when you're hungry, eat what your body needs, stay focused on the food, eliminate distractions (like reading or watching TV) while eating, and pay attention to body cues of hunger and satiety.

Geneen Roth, author of *Women Food and God*, also discusses eating with awareness in her many books and tells her retreat students to "remember two things: to eat what they want when they're hungry and to feel what they feel when they're not." (101). Wow, what powerful words!

In addition, my friend and colleague Sylvia Haskvitz has written a helpful book, *Eat By Choice, Not By Habit*, which uses food, health, and well-being as the portal to the process of nonviolent communication (NVC), which we learned about in chapter 3. She explores underlying needs and shows you how to become reacquainted with the tastes, smells, and sensations of healthful eating.

I hate to say this, but I want to be honest here. Some days, I do just fine with being very mindful about eating when I am hungry and stopping when I am full. My challenge is that I don't quite have a handle on what it feels like in my body to be comfortably full. Therefore, I often use my brain to decide how much to eat (what is a healthy portion?) rather than bodily cues. Jeanne Rust, founder of Mirasol Eating Disorder Recovery Centers, told me that this is the last area to be healed in folks with food-abuse issues. I, too, am still a work in progress!

Some health-conscious people might be touting their new way of eating as being the healthiest and best for everyone. That includes raw foodists, vegetarians, or anyone who strictly follows a specified diet. In his book *Health Food Junkies*, Dr. Steven Bratman coined the term *orthorexia nervosa*, which is characterized by an unhealthy obsession with eating healthy food. Those who have this obsession may:

- make food a moral decision: good versus bad food,
- feel virtuous about their food choices,
- feel critical of those who they perceive as not eating as healthily as they do,
- choose the "right" foods to have the feeling of being in total control,
- eat because of nutritional value or specific ingredients, paying little heed to desires,
- choose to go hungry rather than eat a "forbidden" food,
- isolate, be unable to eat out or attend parties because of dietary restrictions,
- think about food constantly.

This is healthy eating taken to its extreme and is mentioned here as a cautionary note. If you become preoccupied with always eating the "right" food, you may have crossed the line.

Triggers

Just as the newly recovering alcoholic won't step foot into a bar, there may be places and people that you avoid in your newfound recovery from emotional overeating. Please consider the following:

- Are there people in your life who consciously or unconsciously sabotage your efforts? They are the ones who tell you, "Oh, just one bite won't hurt," "You are always on a diet—it's time to live a little," or "I made this specially for you—you have to eat it!" Our support people wouldn't say such things—they want to help us succeed in eliminating the emotional eating. Be very conscious of food pushers, keeping your distance from them if possible.

- Are there specific places that always trigger you to eat more than you want? A restaurant? Your parents' home? Driving past the bakery or Dairy Queen? A buffet filled with your favorite foods and desserts? You can choose to steer clear of these places, or you can find out what is underneath the drive to eat before going and work with yourself around it.

- What are some of your habits around food? When you go to the movie theater, do you always have to get popcorn? When you take a trip, do you always need to have candy in your purse or pocket? When you have your morning coffee, does your mouth seek something sweet at the same time? Do you continually want something in your mouth?

Work on identifying the difference between mouth hunger and stomach hunger. (Mouth hunger is a result of emotional discomfort—chewing, swallowing, and filling up on food can distract from or relieve distress.) Break your unconscious habits, so when you eat it is a conscious decision and not an automatic response.

- Are there certain foods that, once you start eating, you finish the whole thing? Chips, crackers, candy, cookies, and ice cream are among the usual choices. If you can't have a certain something around because you'd eat it all, then don't have it around. As you gain strength and confidence in your new way of binge-free eating, you can gradually reintroduce foods.

- Are you susceptible to TV ads or bulletin boards featuring food? Does the mere sighting of food makes you want to chow down? If so, become aware of your reaction, and if you start drooling during the commercial, change the channel or call your support person. Or how about talking to that part of you that is salivating—what does it really need?

- Does your car automatically pull in to your favorite fast-food drive-through lane? Change your route, avoiding this place if you can. Or find an intervention that works, like calling your buddy as you approach the restaurant.

- H. A. L. T.: Don't let yourself get too Hungry, Angry, Lonely, or Tired—if you do, you are more tempted to eat compulsively:

  When *hungry*, you find it is very easy to grab whatever is convenient and shove it into your mouth. Plan a snack to carry with you when you know there are many hours between meals, so you won't feel ravenous.

  When *angry*, journal, tap, or tell someone about it. Your old way of being is to quickly get your hands on something and wolf it down.

  When *lonely*, move out of isolation (that comfortable, habitual place you go to compulsively overeat) by connecting to someone via phone or email or in person. Move past your loneliness by not being alone, or tap on it, write about it, dialogue with the part of you that is lonely, or intensify your spiritual connection.

  When *tired*, your knee-jerk reaction is to hastily scarf a snack. Sometimes the food does revitalize you; sometimes, though, it causes you to be even more tired. Monitor your energy level, and don't let it drop so low that food seems to be the only solution. Get enough sleep so you won't be tired. Also, this seems silly to say, but I need to hear it for myself—sometimes when you are tired and find yourself seeking something to eat in order to stay awake, the best thing you can really do for yourself is . . . go to sleep!

Stop Eating Your Heart Out

Muscle Testing, or Energy Testing

Muscle testing is a useful technique to discover what your body likes and dislikes. Although a full discussion is beyond the scope of this book, doing an online search for "manual muscle testing" will give you a plethora of information.

My friend and teacher Donna Eden (a phenomenal instructor of energy medicine), uses muscle testing to discover what foods/substances are beneficial, neutral, or detrimental to your body. Energy testing, Donna's name for muscle testing, allows you to determine if the food you are thinking of eating is something your body wants or not. In her book *Energy Medicine* she asserts:

> When the energy of a food, vitamin, or supplement doesn't match the energy of your body, you will not absorb and metabolize it—even if all the experts in the world say you need it. . . . Energy testing can help you know what your body needs at a given moment, and it can help you develop a superb nutrition program for your unique body (61).

Using the *Lean Test*—allowing your body to be used as a pendulum, leaning into or away from the food—is a way to energy test a substance that you want to ingest. Here's how to do it:

Lean Test

Standing straight (with knees soft), ask your body to show you a yes, and then ask it to show you a no. Most people lean forward to indicate yes and backward to indicate no.

Now hold a glass of water to your stomach area. If your body leans forward toward the water, it is favorable (likely purified and free of chlorine and fluoride). If it leans backward away from the water, it is detrimental. And if your body didn't move, the water is neutral.

Test other substances. You might want to start with something easy, in terms of results, like sugar or Splenda. The energy test will most likely show both to be detrimental. Then try a piece of fresh fruit or a vegetable—the energy test will usually show it is beneficial. Make sure you are in a relaxed stance with the knees slightly bent so you can feel the movement forward or backward. Some people feel only a tiny movement; with others, their whole body rocks forward or backward.

◆

You can choose to energy test any and all foods. The choice is yours. Have a clear intent as you hold the substance, asking, "Is this beneficial for my body now?" I often energy test my foods, choosing many advantageous and neutral foods and staying away from the unfavorable ones. Doing so increases my health and vitality. Neglecting this and choosing foods that are detrimental often causes me to lose energy and clarity and sometimes even gives me a bellyache. Once you get the hang of this, you won't need to have the actual food in front of you—just the listing of it on a menu is sometimes enough.

Assignment

Identify triggers for yourself. List people, places, situations, and events that might trigger you to eat compulsively. Next to each, write down a possible remedy or solution.

It is important to pay attention to the effect food and meals have on your energy level. Before you eat your next meal, write down your energy level (with 10 being the highest). Monitor your energy. Is it higher, lower, or the same right after the meal? Thirty minutes later? An hour later? With this information, you now have a choice: *Do I choose to eat _____ [specific food] even though my energy level may decrease?* In addition, to keep your energy high and balanced, you can choose to energy test any and all food before you consume it.

Most people find that their energy is higher and more balanced the more they choose natural, unprocessed foods—fruits, vegetables, nuts, seeds, etc. And the more they eat processed foods (especially white flour and sugar), the more they pay a price energetically, by feeling tired and lethargic.

Plan a conscious eating experience for yourself. Be seated in a quiet, peaceful spot. Eat only when you are hungry and focus on the food—the tastes, smells, and textures. Avoid distractions (no watching TV or listening to the radio, no talking on the phone, no reading), so you can totally concentrate on the activity of eating. Eat what your body wants and stop when you are not totally full. Savor the food and enjoy the experience.

Chapter 9

Putting It All Together

*What the caterpillar calls the end of the world,
the master calls a butterfly.*
—RICHARD BACH, *ILLUSIONS*

WHEW! YOU MADE IT THROUGH. Twenty-one days of assignments to give you a slew of new tools to end your emotional eating! When you first started this journey with me, you took a little quiz to determine whether you were a compulsive overeater or not. Let's take the quiz again, noting the ones that apply to you all or much of the time:

- I am preoccupied with food, eating, and weight.
- I am aware that my eating patterns are not normal.
- I eat when I am not physically hungry.
- I eat very little in public and binge in private.
- I eat to comfort myself and relieve distressing feelings.
- I tend to eat more when I am stressed, anxious, or depressed.

- I graze all day, often needing something in my mouth.
- Food has become my friend, my lover, or my drug of choice.
- I sometimes feel hungry even after a large meal.
- I eat more rapidly than other people.
- I allow the scale to determine if I have a good or bad day.
- I eat until my stomach hurts or I feel nauseated.
- I feel ashamed of myself due to the quantity of food I consume.
- I feel powerless over my eating behavior.
- I eat before I go to bed at night so I can sleep.
- I use food as a reward.
- I eat when I am bored, tired, or feeling blah.
- I eat when I see food ads on TV.
- I often stop to get fast food and eat it in the car.
- I am secretive about what I eat and how much I eat.
- I eagerly anticipate the times I can eat alone.
- I am an overachiever and want to be in control.
- I often think I am worthless or not good enough.
- I frequently compare my body size to that of others.
- I make derogatory jokes about my eating or body size.
- I have tried many diets, unsuccessfully.
- I am terrified that I will keep gaining weight.

Now, compare this list with the one you completed in chapter 2, when you first started to address your compulsive overeating. Are fewer of these true for you now that you have progressed on this adventure of ending the emotional eating? If the number is the same, don't be disheartened—this is a process, and your progress will soon be observable. Once in a while a few clients have reported more items are true for them this time through the list. When we discuss how that could be, they realize that they had not been completely truthful the first time through and that doing the assignments has led them to a new level of self-honesty.

In addition to the items that are no longer true for you on this list, are you aware of other changes you have made? Not giving in, perhaps, every time you are tempted to compulsively overeat? Choosing food for nutrition rather than for the sugar or fat satisfaction? Feeling better about yourself? Having hope that this time really is different? Being able to look in the mirror and see a wonderful, beautiful person smiling back at you? As you consistently use your new tools, you will continue to evolve and your eating behavior and your relationship with food will also continue to change.

Let's recap and discuss how you might want to use the tools you've learned over the past 21 days on an ongoing basis:

Day 1: Eating History. When you wrote your eating history as your first assignment, you were just getting started. Since then, you may have had other memories surface about your eating behaviors that you can add to your written account. The purpose of the assignment was for you to get honest with yourself about how you've used food in the past. Hold on to what you wrote, so you can remind yourself what it used to be like for you. Add to it whenever other memories bring you additional details.

Day 2: Food-Mood Diary. For many of us emotional overeaters, it will take some time to really connect our experiences and our feelings with what we pop into our mouths. It is a good idea to continue writing your food-feelings connections to give you more and more insights and awareness. When you write down every tidbit that you eat, there is less chance of unconsciously nibbling on something since you have the task of writing it down. Also, because you now have the tapping tools, you can intervene immediately and not grab for the food when the craving hits.

Day 3: Personal Journal. Writing is a great tool to continue to use—it allows you to expand on your thoughts and often encourages additional ones to emerge. We who used to eat over our feelings can now allow ourselves to experience them, write about them, and come to terms with them—we know they won't destroy us. As you write, are you gaining a greater understanding of your eating behavior, your thoughts and beliefs? Have you noticed that sometimes your beliefs are not based in reality?

Stop Eating Your Heart Out

Many of our beliefs are untrue, unrealistic, or just plain nonsense. When we are convinced of these beliefs, we end up with negative feelings that add to our anxiety, depression, and food compulsion. Byron Katie teaches in her book *Loving What Is: Four Questions That Can Change Your Life*:

> Whenever we experience a stressful feeling—anything from mild discomfort to intense sorrow, rage, or despair—we can be certain that there is a specific thought causing our reaction, whether or not we are conscious of it. The way to end our stress is to investigate the thinking that lies behind it (ix).

As you read through your journal and food-mood diary, take on the role of observer and use the process of inquiry. Because thoughts and beliefs can create your suffering, begin to question those thoughts and beliefs and the meanings you have given them.

Day 4: Creating a Support System. Have you found a buddy to accompany you on your journey? If you are attending a Twelve-Step support group, you should have a sponsor, I hope. Whatever your support system, if it feels right and is giving you the assistance you want, stay with it. If not, search out another type of support group or additional supportive friends to encourage you.

Day 5: Self-Care. Keep up the daily activity of nurturing yourself. You deserve it! Continue to monitor your thoughts and words, so that when you hear yourself mutter, "I have to," change it to "I choose to." In addition, replace each *should* with *could*. Modifying your thoughts and words continues to keep you in a place of empowerment and out of victim thinking.

Day 6: Therapy. Perhaps you are now seeing a psychotherapist—continue for as long as necessary. If you are not seeing a therapist, remember that this is always an option to help you in your growth and healing, so keep it in the back of your mind.

Day 7: Higher Power. You are spending time each day connecting with and deepening your relationship to your Higher Power. Keep it up. Changing your relationship with food is a big undertaking, and strengthening your spiritual connection helps a great deal.

Day 8: Prayer and Meditation. Are you beginning and ending each day with prayer? Please continue to do so. Are you meditating at least once a day? You can use the same type of meditation, or you can experiment with different ones; the important element is doing something spiritual on a daily basis. Remember, as the prayer and meditation increases, the food compulsion decreases because you are being filled in a different way.

Day 9: Creative Visualization. Whenever you want, you can do a creative visualization or create a vision board to solidify your dreams and goals and help in the manifestation of them. Continue to see (and feel) yourself enjoying a new relationship with food: No longer driven to compulsively overeat, you are now eating for pleasure and nutrition.

Day 10: An Introduction to TFT and EFT. I hope you are using EFT any time you need to quell the awfulness of a feeling. Remember, when a distressing emotion arises, tapping brings down the charge and extinguishes the need to abuse food. Sometimes, instead of actually tapping, you can use your imagination and visualize tapping on the points.

Day 11: Rapidly Integrated Transformation Technique (RITT). Like EFT, RITT decreases the intensity of overpowering emotions, so those feelings will not compel you to eat/overeat/binge. Also, both RITT and EFT are extremely effective in curbing cravings—when you think of wolfing something down, use RITT or EFT to mitigate the urge. Try this: Think about a food craving. Shut your eyes and really feel yourself having this intense desire. Take a few deep breaths. Where do you feel it in your body? What are your thoughts? Now, allow yourself to go deeper—what is the need beneath those thoughts and feelings? If you're thinking "I just want it," then keep digging. Are you feeling lonely? Tired? Annoyed? Anxious? What is it you are really seeking? Once you have identified underlying feelings, use EFT or RITT. As the tapping diminishes the intensity of the feelings, the obsession lifts.

Day 12: Personal Energy Work. Have you been monitoring your energy level and identifying energizers and drains? When your energy falls, there is a tendency to reach for food, so keeping it high and balanced helps you in the achievement of freedom from emotional eating. When you are with difficult people or experiencing challenging situations, remember to send or channel Universal energy to keep your own personal energy elevated. What are your favorite quick-energy pick-me-ups? Keep on using these techniques as needed.

Day 13: The Inner Child. I hope you have been taking on the role of the Healthy Adult and conversing with your Inner Child. Often it is the child (or the rebellious adolescent) part of us that is actually reaching for something to eat, and dialoguing helps you to understand and change that behavior. Connect with your Inner Child to continue to heal your past. Dr. Hew Len refers to that part as the subconscious, and he believes we must continue to heal that aspect for our personal benefit, as well as to help heal the world.

Day 14: Right-Hand/Left-Hand Dialogue. Using this technique enables you to work with subconscious parts.

You can use it with the Inner Child as well as with other parts of yourself (your back that hurts, for instance, or the part of you that feels lonely). If a certain food keeps calling you, this technique might help you discover the causative feelings and needs.

Day 15: Parts Work—Embracing the Inner Critic. Have you been able to identify the voice of the Inner Critic without succumbing to it? There are several ways to do parts work: Chair Work, Two Hands Talking, and Right-Hand/Left-Hand Dialogue. Continue to use whatever methods you like.

Day 16: Mini Inventory. It is important to keep on monitoring your behaviors by taking a daily mini inventory. Before you go to sleep each night, review your day. Are there people you spoke to harshly? Do you wish you would have said or done something differently? The goal is to observe your behavior without judgment and be immediately accountable. Owning all your behaviors (with self-compassion) derails the food cravings.

Day 17: Giving It Away. When you uncover additional character defects, it is a good idea to write about them and discuss them with a confidante. This action might only be necessary on occasion.

Day 18: Making Amends. After you have reviewed your day (Day 16) and discovered you wish you had acted or spoken differently, make direct amends as soon as possible to those whom you identified as having harmed. Then the need for amends won't pile up —you take care of them as soon as you discover they are needed. Again, the more you take responsibility by making amends and changing behaviors, the less often food calls your name.

Day 19: Forgiveness. When you reviewed your day (Day 16), you may have found that you need to ask someone for forgiveness. Do so as soon as possible. When you act out of integrity and catch yourself doing something "wrong," you are able to ask for forgiveness immediately. Continue to ask in your daily meditation, "Who do I need to forgive today?" Do you still need to forgive yourself? In addition, remember to use Ho'oponopono.

Day 20: Gratitude. Each evening, remember to think of at least one thing you are grateful for. When you are feeling down, write a gratitude list—or do it anytime the notion strikes you. Remind yourself to reframe events, seeking the silver lining. The more you are living in a state of appreciation, the more food is just food, rather than your drug of choice.

Day 21 Healthy Eating. Keep monitoring your triggers and be aware of H. A. L. T. (don't get too hungry, angry, lonely, or tired). Energy test your food some or all of the time. Pay attention to how you feel and what your energy level is when you eat. Increase the number of meals when you practice conscious eating.

◆

Now that you have a mighty full toolbox, let's take a look at how you might use it as you continue to break old habits and rewire your brain. Here are some typical scenarios:

Situation: You come home from work tired and ravenous.

Old Response: Stop for fast food or grab the first thing you see in the refrigerator.

Other Options:
- Plan ahead and have a snack available so you are not famished.
- Meditate or sit and breathe for a few minutes.
- Call your buddy/support person.

Situation: The kids are in bed, spouse is out, and you want to indulge in your favorite snack food.

Old Response: Turn on the TV, kick back, and mindlessly munch, munch, munch!

Other Options:
- Dialogue with that part that wants the food. What are the real needs?

- Have the snack food if you want, but focus on it with the TV off.
- Journal.

Situation: You are worried or feeling anxious.

Old Response: Indulge in a high-fat/high-sugar treat.

Other Options:
- Tap on the anxiety.
- Call a friend/support person.
- Meditate or sit and breathe for a few minutes.

Situation: You are feeling tired, though it is still an hour or two before bedtime.

Old Response: Seek out a treat to feel re-energized.

Other Options:
- Do an energy pick-me-up.
- Engage in a self-nurturing activity, such as taking a bubble bath or reading.
- Go to bed early!

Situation: You had a fight or disagreement with someone close.

Old Response: Grab something to eat and stuff it in.

Other Options:
- Tap.
- Journal.
- Call your buddy/support person.

Situation: The old "I don't care" voice is pulling you back to old habits with food.

Old Response: Give the voice free reign and do whatever it wants.

Other Options:
- Do parts work to determine what the needs are beneath the words.
- Do Inner Child work or Right-Hand/Left-Hand Dialogue.
- Do a creative visualization where you imagine yourself free of emotional eating.

Situation: Your favorite snack food is screaming your name.

Old Response: You eat it rapidly, sometimes gorging yourself.

Other Options:
- Tap.
- Right-Hand/Left-Hand Dialogue—what is going on underneath?
- Self-nurture with an activity from your list.

Situation: You are at a party and there is a ton of junk food.

Old Response: Eat, eat, eat. (If you were a secret binger, you might eat a little at a time and keep going back for more.)

Other Options:

- Tap. (You can successfully do this in your imagination.)

- Call a support person.

- Go into the restroom and spend a few minutes breathing/centering/praying.

Situation: You pass a fast-food place and deceive yourself into thinking you are just going to get a drink or a salad or something little to tide you over.

Old Response: Order and eat way too much.

Other Options:

- Don't stop at the fast-food joint!

- Call your buddy/support person.

- If you end up buying the burger and fries, eat slowly and really taste the food.

Situation: You are feeling bored and have nothing to do.

Old Response: Head to the fridge for a snack.

Other Options:
- Write a gratitude list.
- Engage in a self-nurturing activity.
- Reread this book.

These are merely suggestions for some typical occurrences. When a situation comes up, open your toolbox and use whatever tool feels right for the moment. Sometimes you may try one and find it doesn't work—then proceed to try out another and another.

One day when I was feeling glum, I tried using several different tools: Talking with my Inner Child didn't lift my mood, tapping didn't change it either, and even dialoguing with the dejected part of me didn't work. Spontaneously, I made up a little ditty and began a sort of singing chant:

I love my life. I love my life.
I love my life, oh yes, I do.
Oh, I love my life. I love my life.
I love my life. Yes, indeed I do.

As fast as snapping my fingers, I felt better. Instead of feeling grumpy, I now felt happy and energized. Somehow, the words plus the vibration of the tune worked in lifting my spirits.

My suggestion to you is to experiment with all the tools you've been given. If none seem to be working in the moment, go outside the (tool)box. Be creative. Persevere. You are the master of your life and the interventionist who can find a solution to your predicament or change your disposition.

Bonus Technique #1: WHEE

On my quest for being the best me I can be, I persist in exploring additional personal-growth methods. Although you've already experienced twenty-one days of assignments and tools, here is another easy one for you to try and add to your toolbox as a bonus!

Sometimes I want a tapping technique that's quicker than EFT or RITT, so I work with WHEE (Whole Health Easily and Effectively), a hybrid of EMDR (Eve Movement Desensitization and Reprocessing) and EFT. Dr. Daniel Benor, a holistic psychiatric psychotherapist, had only very brief sessions with each patient, and he needed a quick and uncomplicated treatment. So he developed WHEE, which is basically stimulating the right and left sides of the body while repeating an affirmation. It is easy to learn and easy to do—try it for yourself:

1. Think of an issue that brings up emotional discomfort. Rate the charge or discomfort using the 0–10 scale, with 10 being the most intense.

2. Now give yourself a bear hug. That's right; hug yourself, placing your right hand on your upper left arm and your left hand on your upper right

Stop Eating Your Heart Out

arm. It's also known as a "butterfly hug." Think of your issue and say, "Even though I am feeling _____ , I totally love and accept myself." Continue repeating the words as you alternate tapping your upper arms—tap with your right hand, then your left hand. Right, left, right, left. Keep going for a few minutes.

3. Stop and take a breath.

4. Think back to your original issue and now rate the level of emotional discomfort.

5. If the number is higher than 1, repeat this process until the feelings have dissipated.

Check out *www.paintap.com* for a detailed protocol. When I am in a hurry, I often use WHEE, with great results. My clients, too, have found this method to be easy and effective.

Bonus Technique #2: Inner-Work Walks

Most every day my dog Sadie and I walk the arroyo near my house, combining exercise with inner work. I refer to these walks as my Inner-Work Walks. I began doing this when I was doing a liver cleanse; I decided since I was cleaning out my physical insides, I also wanted to clean out my emotional insides (by identifying core beliefs and re-parenting my Inner Child).

Although I am no longer on a liver cleanse, I continue to connect with my Child Within on these walks as an important part of my ongoing personal-growth work. Because I desire to eliminate excess weight, I check in with all my inner children, all my parts, to see if they are in agreement or if they have specific needs. It is amazing—whenever an issue comes up and I find a way to resolve it, I am able to drop some weight again. For instance, when I once asked if any parts didn't want me to lose more weight, an adolescent voice identified herself. She was worried I'd be too sexy, and she felt scared. My Nurturing Parent part reassured her and then imagined her encased in a blue-white light. She smiled and okayed more weight loss—and I was able to release another two pounds.

I have found that this works for me—please discover for yourself what works for you. If these Inner-Work Walks feel right for you, then go ahead and add them to your day. If not, find a way to continue doing your inner work. Maybe you have alone time each morning or evening. Maybe you take a whole day once a week to focus totally on you and your recovery from emotional eating.

Conclusion

I came into Twelve-Step Recovery thinking I was damaged goods. I saw myself as a fraud—always appearing to be calm, cool, and collected. Inside, though, I was numb most of the time. Babies experience what is sometimes called a milk coma—after eating, they drift peacefully off to sleep. I felt as if I often experienced a food coma, but it wasn't as pleasant as the milk coma sounded. It did keep me deadened and in a sort of stupor, with a smile plastered on.

Inside I was crying. But that was way inside, and I did my best to not touch that place—the pit deep within, filled with despair.

Like the butterfly spending the first part of its life in a chrysalis, I too spent my early years in hiding, keeping myself separate from others. Joining a Twelve-Step support group was the beginning of my metamorphosis. I am not the person I was when I began my journey of recovery as a twenty-nine-year-young woman. Gone is the self-absorbed, superior-acting woman who felt like a screwed-up hypocrite. Gone is the binge eater. Gone is the timid woman always seeking another's approval. In her place is a woman of substance, not weight. A woman who knows her worth and assists others in finding theirs. A woman who chooses healthy eating and, instead of licking her plate clean, has licked her binge eating disorder.

Although you and I have probably not met in person, if you are anything like me, I know you. You may have been in hiding a long time, too, but now that you have come face-to-face with your food and eating issues, you are growing and changing and getting healthier. I know, too, that you are unique, that you have many talents to share, and that you are, in the eyes of the Divine, perfect just the way you are.

My wish is that this book has made a contribution in exposing you to the real you and has assisted you in changing your relationship not only with food but also with yourself. You opened this book to end your food obsession and, in doing the assignments, you discovered the journey is really all about personal growth and uncovering your true Self. As you continue evolving, my desire for you is that you appreciate the total you and your specialness. Just like the caterpillar, you are in the process of transformation. And, as you emerge from the darkness of emotional overeating, you, too, will soar.

Epilogue
· · · · · · · · · ·

We must embrace pain and burn it as fuel for our journey.

—Kenji Miyazawa, Japanese poet

I FINISHED EDITING THIS BOOK'S manuscript around 6 PM EDT on October 12, 2011. Little did I know that at approximately the same time Jonathan, my sweet, loving, thirty-five-year-old son was finishing too: two thousand miles away, he pulled the trigger that ended his life.

I was devastated. Shocked. Angry. Grief-stricken. Heartbroken. Raw.

How have I coped with this enormous loss and excruciating pain without the old crutch of compulsive overeating? I have used the tools presented here, over and over again: allowing myself to feel and discharge my feelings; crying and weeping, some days a lot, some days a little; tapping using EFT, RITT, and WHEE; praying and meditating; leaning on my support people; asking my spiritual family to send me energy; doing parts work; journaling; recognizing and working with the Inner Critic; forgiving myself and Jon; making amends (again, myself and Jon);

doing Ho'oponopono; trying to laugh at least once a day; focusing, in gratitude, on the thirty-five years Jon was with us; choosing (mostly) healthy eating; and sometimes, just sitting and remembering to breathe.

In addition, I have been reading many books about what happens after we die, about our soul's destiny and plans, and about losing a child. Danielle Steel lost her nineteen-year-old son to suicide and wrote (on the back cover of Suzanne Redfern and Susan K. Gilbert's *The Grieving Garden: Living with the Death of a Child*):

> There is no right or wrong way to grieve. Each person must find the way that makes sense and works for them, in a situation that makes no sense. Losing a child is nine parts unthinkably horrible, and one part gift. The secret to surviving it is finding the gift. One is never the same, but one has the choice of becoming bigger, deeper, more.

Seeking to find the gift, the silver lining, I am comforted in my belief that it will come in time. I am pleasantly surprised at my attitude: I don't want to waste the pain, it is here and I can't escape it; therefore, I choose to use it for my growth. To do so, I must continue using all the tools at my disposal so I won't lose myself to the pain and morbidity. Instead, I intend to come through this stronger, with my heart more fully opened, and more divinely connected than before. It is my hope that you too can not only survive whatever difficulties life throws at you without emotional eating, but will also use those challenges for your own personal growth.

There is a sacredness in tears. They are not the mark of weakness, but of power. They speak more eloquently than ten thousand tongues. They are messengers of overwhelming grief…and unspeakable love.

—Washington Irving, American author

To read more about Jon and my process around his passing, please visit *www.jonathanhersheybeck.com*.

—Meryl, 12-12-11 (2 months after Jon's passing)

Daily Assignments Overview
. . . .

1. **Eating History.** Writing your past use of food; discussing your relationship with food.
2. **Food-Mood Diary.** Logging your food and moods every time you eat.
3. **Personal Journal.** Writing every day; seeking to discover and work with your feelings.
4. **Creating a Support System.** Finding a support group, a buddy, and supportive people.
5. **Self-Care.** Finding ways to nurture yourself. Eliminating the *shoulds* and *have tos.*
6. **Therapy.** Exploring whether or not you want to see a psychotherapist at this time.
7. **Higher Power.** Strengthening your spiritual connection; write a letter to your Higher Power and link in to a Loving Presence every day.
8. **Prayer and Meditation.** Daily praying and meditating. Any type, your choice.
9. **Creative Visualization.** Seeing yourself free from emotional eating, and perhaps creating a vision board, too.
10. **An Introduction to TFT and EFT.** Using EFT to eliminate uncomfortable feelings.

11. **Rapidly Integrated Transformation Technique (RITT).** Using RITT to quell food cravings.

12. **Personal Energy Work.** Monitoring your energy. Sending energy. Identifying energizers and drains. Using energy pick-me-ups.

13. **The Inner Child.** Finding/creating the Healthy Adult. Connecting to the precious child you once were.

14. **Right-Hand/Left-Hand Dialogue.** Using both hands to dialogue with your Inner Child or with different parts of yourself.

15. **Parts Work.** Identifying the Inner Critic voice, and embracing the Inner Critic. Using parts work— Chair Work and Two Hands Talking.

16. **Mini Inventory.** Writing about past wrongs and the Seven Deadly Sins.

17. **Giving It Away.** Sharing with your Higher Power and also a confidant what you wrote on Day 16.

18. **Making Amends.** Admitting your mistakes, asking for forgiveness, rectifying the situation, and changing the behaviors.

19. **Forgiveness.** Releasing old resentments and forgiving those who have harmed you.

20. **Gratitude.** Writing a gratitude list; reframing events as you look for the silver linings.

21. **Healthy Eating.** Identifying triggers. Energy testing your food. Choosing conscious eating and non-processed food as much as possible.

Resources

. . . .

THERE ARE A MULTITUDE OF support groups and resources available to compulsive overeaters and their families. And some, like NVC and RA, are open to everyone.

NVC—Nonviolent Communication is based on the principles of nonviolence—the natural state of compassion when no violence is present in the heart. NVC practice groups can now be found in over forty countries. *www.cnvc.org*

Twelve-Step Groups

ABA—Anorexics and Bulimics Anonymous is a fellowship that believes eating disorders are about an illusion of control over food and body weight. The only requirement for membership is a desire to stop unhealthy eating practices. *www.aba12steps.org*

CEA—Compulsive Eaters Anonymous is a fellowship of individuals who, through shared experience, strength, and hope, are recovering from compulsive eating and food addiction. They welcome everyone who wants to stop eating compulsively. *www.ceahow.org*

EAA—Eating Addictions Anonymous is a fellowship of people recovering from all aspects of eating addiction and body obsession. Since food is but a symptom, they do not believe lasting recovery can be based on any particular plan of eating, but only by a thorough working of the Twelve Steps. *www.eatingaddictionsanonymous.org*

EDA—Eating Disorders Anonymous is a fellowship of individuals who share their experience, strength, and hope with each other that they may solve their common problems and help others recover from their eating disorders. EDA endorses sound nutrition and discourages any form of rigidity around food. *www.eatingdisordersanonymous.org*

FAA—Food Addicts Anonymous is an organization that believes that food addiction is a biochemical disorder that occurs at a cellular level and therefore cannot be cured by willpower or by therapy alone. This Twelve-Step Program believes that food addiction can be managed by eliminating addictive foods, following a program of sound nutrition, and working the Twelve Steps of the program. *www.foodaddictsanonymous.org*

FA—Food Addicts in Recovery Anonymous is an international fellowship of men and women who have experienced difficulties in life as a result of the way they eat. Membership is open to anyone who wants help with food. *www.foodaddicts.org*

GSA—GreySheeters Anonymous was founded and designed to discuss the fundamentals or basics of attaining and maintaining GreySheet abstinence, which they define as three weighed and measured meals a day from a specific food plan—the GreySheet—with nothing in between but black coffee, tea, or diet soda. *www.greysheet.org*

OA—Overeaters Anonymous offers a program of recovery from compulsive eating using the Twelve Steps and Twelve Traditions of OA. It addresses physical, emotional, and spiritual well-being. It is not a religious organization and does not promote any particular diet. *www.oa.org*

RA—Recoveries Anonymous is a Solution Focused Twelve Step program. RA is open to everyone, not just those with food issues. *www.r-a.org*

Online Resources

Academy for Eating Disorders is a global professional association committed to leadership in eating disorders research, education, treatment, and prevention.
www.aedweb.org
(847) 498-4274

The Alliance for Eating Disorders Awareness conveys the message that recovery from eating disorders is possible, and that individuals should not have to suffer or recover alone.
www.allianceforeatingdisorders.com
(866) 662-1235

Am I Hungry? teaches intuitive eating to end yo-yo dieting.
www.amihungry.org
(480) 704-7811

Binge Eating Disorder Association (BEDA) was founded to help those who have binge eating disorder, their friends and family, and those who treat the disorder.
www.bedaonline.org
(855) 855-2323

The Body Image Project focuses on reframing body image and features weekly stories from real people discussing their body image struggles and triumphs.
www.bodyimageproject.com

Eating-Disorder-Information.com provides information on all the eating disorders.
www.eating-disorder-information.com

Eating Disorder Recovery is a site created by Joanna Poppink, a psychotherapist and author specializing in eating disorder recovery for adult women and the challenges women face after recovery as they rebuild their lives.
www.eatingdisorderrecovery.com

Eating Disorder Referral and Information Center
is dedicated to the prevention and treatment of eating
disorders and offers a comprehensive database of eating
disorder treatment professionals.
www.edreferral.com
(858) 792-7463

Eating Disorders Coalition seeks to advance the federal
recognition of eating disorders as a public health priority.
www.eatingdisorderscoalition.org
(202) 543-9570

Eating Disorders Information Network (EDIN) is
committed to the prevention of all types of disordered
eating and the promotion of positive body-esteem
through education, outreach, and action.
www.myedin.org
(404) 816-3346

Eating Disorders Online.com offers support, news,
and pathways to treatment.
www.eatingdisordersonline.com
(310) 476-4924

Eating Disorders Treatment provides information
and resources.
www.eating-disorder.com
(866) 575-8179

The Gail R. Schoenbach F.R.E.E.D. Foundation is a nonprofit organization dedicated to eradicating eating disorders. The funds contributed to the F.R.E.E.D. Foundation provide individuals the financial support needed for the treatment of eating disorders.
www.freedfoundation.org

Health at Every Size (HAES) is based on the simple premise that the best way to improve health is to honor your body. It supports people in adopting health habits for the sake of health and well-being (rather than weight control).
www.haescommunity.org

Healthy Girl is an online support site for girls and young women who binge or emotionally overeat.
www.healthygirl.org

The Original Intuitive Eating Pros website offers a multitude of resources to create a healthy relationship with food, mind, and body.
www.intuitiveeating.org
(310) 551-1999

MentorConnect is designed to replace eating disorders with relationships; it is the first global, online pro-recovery eating disorders mentoring community and provides one-on-one mentoring matches for individuals seeking recovery.
www.mentorconnect-ed.org

National Association for Males with Eating Disorders (N.A.M.E.D.) is dedicated to offering support and public awareness about males with eating disorders.
www.namedinc.org
(877) 780-0080

National Association of Anorexia Nervosa and Associated Disorders (ANAD) is a nonprofit dedicated to the prevention and alleviation of eating disorders.
www.anad.org
(630) 577-1333

The National Eating Disorder Information Centre (NEDIC) is a Canadian nonprofit organization that provides information and resources on eating disorders and weight preoccupation.
www.nedic.ca
(866) 633-4220

National Eating Disorders Association (NEDA) supports individuals and families affected by eating disorders, and serves as a catalyst for prevention, cures and access to quality care.
www.nationaleatingdisorders.org
(206) 382-3587

Stop Eating Your Heart Out

National Eating Disorders Screening Program (NED-SP) represents the first large-scale screening for eating disorders.
www.nmisp.org
(781) 239-0071

Something Fishy is dedicated to raising awareness and providing support for people with eating disorders and has a directory of treatment providers and support groups.
www.something-fishy.org
(866) 690-7239

Eating Disorder Treatment Centers

There are residential as well as outpatient treatment centers in the United States and around the world that offer help for compulsive overeating and binge eating disorder. Here are a few of the many treatment centers. Check out *www.edreferral.com* for a more complete list or talk to your health care provider.

The Bella Vita
www.thebellavita.com
(818) 585-1775

Bodywise Binge Eating Recovery Program
www.stopcompulsiveeating.com
(888) 371-0671

Castlewood Treatment Center for Eating Disorders
www.castlewoodtc.com
(888) 822-8938

Center for Change
www.centerforchange.com
(888) 224-8250

Columbia University Medical Center/New York
Offers free residential treatment for as much as four months if the individual is willing to be part of ongoing research.
www.cumc.columbia.edu
(212) 305-CUMC

Cottonwood de Tucson

www.cottonwooddetucson.com

(800) 877-4520

Desert Milagros

www.desertmilagros.net

(520) 531-1040

The Emily Program

www.emilyprogram.com

(888) EMILY77

Mirasol is a holistic treatment emphasizing therapies to address underlying stress and trauma. I have visited and spoken with staff and patients—it is a warm, caring atmosphere.

www.mirasol.net

(888) 520-1700

Oliver-Pyatt Centers

www.oliverpyattcenters.com

(866) 511-4325

Rader Programs

www.raderprograms.com

(800) 841-1515

Remuda Ranch

www.remudaranch.com

(888) 527-8205

The Renfrew Center
www.renfrewcenter.com
(800) RENFREW

Sierra Tucson
www.sierratucson.com
(800) 842-4487

Structure House
www.structurehouse.com
(800) 553-0052

University of North Carolina Eating Disorders Program
www.psychiatry.unc.edu/eatingdisorders
(919) 966-7012

Walden Behavioral Care
www.waldenbehavioralcare.com
(781) 647-6727

Recommended Reading

A., Jim. *Recovery from Compulsive Eating: A Complete Guide to the Twelve Step Program.* Center City, MN: Hazelden, 1994.

Albers, Susan. *50 Ways to Soothe Yourself without Food.* Oakland, CA: New Harbinger Publications, 2009.

Alcoholics Anonymous (The Big Book). 4th ed. New York: Alcoholics Anonymous World Services, 2001.

Beattie, Melody. *The Language of Letting Go: Daily Meditations for Codependents.* New York: HarperCollins, 1990.

Beck, Meryl Hershey. "Choices for Weight Control and Stress Management." *Arizona Choices*: Health, Wellness, & the Environment, Feb.–Mar. 2006.

Benor, Daniel J. *Seven Minutes to Natural Pain Release: WHEE for Tapping your Pain Away.* Santa Rosa, CA: Energy Psychology Press, 2008.

Benson, Herbert. *Beyond the Relaxation Response: How to Harness the Power of Your Personal Beliefs.* New York: Berkley Books, 1985.

Booth, Leo. *When God Becomes a Drug.* New York: J.P. Tarcher, 1991.

Borysenko, Joan. *Minding the Body, Mending the Mind*. New York: Bantam, 1988.

Bradshaw, John. *Healing the Shame that Binds You*. Deerfield Beach, FL: Health Communications, 1988.

Bratman, Steven. *Health Food Junkies: Overcoming the Obsession with Healthful Eating*. New York: Broadway Books, 2000.

Bry, Adelaide, and Marjorie Bair. *Directing the Movies of your Mind: Visualization for Health and Insight*. New York: Harper & Row, 1978.

Bulik, Cynthia M. *Crave: Why You Binge Eat and How to Stop*. New York: Walker & Co., 2009.

Buscaglia, Leo F. *Loving Each Other: The Challenge of Human Relationships*. New York: Fawcett Columbine, 1984.

Campos, Paul F. *The Obesity Myth: Why America's Obsession with Weight Is Hazardous to Your Health*. New York: Gotham Books, 2004.

Capacchione, Lucia. *Lighten up Your Body, Lighten up Your Life: Beyond Diet and Exercise—The Inner Path to Lasting Change*. North Hollywood, CA: Newcastle Publishing, 1990.

———. *Recovery of Your Inner Child*. New York: Simon & Schuster, 1991.

Casey, Karen. *A Life of My Own*. Center City, MN: Hazelden, 1993.

Church, Dawson. *The Genie in Your Genes: Epigenetic Medicine and the New Biology of Intention*. Santa Rosa, CA: Elite Books, 2007.

Cohen, Alan. *A Deep Breath of Life: Daily Inspiration for Heart-Centered Living*. Carlsbad, CA: Hay House, 1996.

Craig, Gary. *EFT for Weight Loss*. Santa Rosa, CA: Energy Psychology Press, 2010.

———. *The EFT Manual*. 2nd ed. Santa Rosa, CA: Energy Psychology Press, 2011.

Dyer, Wayne. *Excuses Begone! How to Change Lifelong, Self-Defeating Thinking Habits*. 4th ed. Carlsbad, CA: Hay House, 2011.

Eden, Donna, and David Feinstein. *Energy Medicine: Balancing Your Body's Energies for Optimal Health, Joy, and Vitality*. Updated and expanded ed. New York: Jeremy P. Tarcher/Penguin, 2008.

Emmons, Robert A., and Michael E. McCullough, ed. *The Psychology of Gratitude*. New York: Oxford University Press, 2004.

Epstein, Gerald. *Healing Visualizations: Creating Health through Imagery*. New York: Bantam Books, 1989.

Fairburn, Christopher G. *Overcoming Binge Eating*. New York: Guilford Press, 1995.

Feinstein, David. *Energy Psychology Interactive Self-help Guide*. Ashland, OR: Innersource, 2003.

Feinstein, David, Donna Eden, and Gary Craig. *The Promise of Energy Psychology: Revolutionary Tools for Dramatic Personal Change*. New York: Jeremy P. Tarcher/Penguin, 2005.

Fishel, Ruth. *Time for Joy: Daily Affirmations*. Deerfield Beach, FL: Health Communications, 1988.

Gawain, Shakti. *Creative Visualization: Use the Power of Your Imagination to Create What You Want in Your Life*. 25th anniversary ed. Novato, CA: Nataraj Publishing, 2002.

Gold, Sunny Sea. *Food: The Good Girl's Drug: How to Stop Using Food to Control Your Feelings*. New York: Berkley Books, 2011.

Haskvitz, Sylvia. *Eat by Choice, Not by Habit*. Encinitas, CA: Puddledancer, 2005.

Hay, Louise L. *You Can Heal Your Life*. Carlsbad, CA: Hay House, 1987.

Hirschmann, Jane R., and Carol H. Munter. *When Women Stop Hating Their Bodies: Freeing Yourself from Food and Weight Obsession*. New York: Fawcett Columbine, 1995.

John-Roger, *The Way Out Book*. Los Angeles, CA: Mandeville Press, 1980.

Katherine, Anne. *Anatomy of a Food Addiction*. 3rd ed. Carlsbad, CA: Gurze, 1996.

Katie, Byron, and Stephen Mitchell. *Loving What Is: Four Questions that Can Change Your Life*. New York: Three Rivers Press, 2002.

Kolata, Gina. *Rethinking Thin: The New Science of Weight Loss—and the Myths and Realities of Dieting*. New York: Farrar, Straus, and Giroux, 2007.

Kramer, Dorothea, and Karilee Halo Shames. *Energetic Approaches to Emotional Healing*. Albany, NY: Delmar Publishers, 1997.

L., Elizabeth. *Food for Thought: Daily Meditations for Overeaters*. 2nd ed. Center City, MN: Hazelden, 1992.

Larsen, Earnie, and Carol Hegarty. *Believing in Myself: Daily Meditations for Healing and Building Self-Esteem*. New York: Fireside/Parkside, 1991.

Loweree, Frank H. *The 12 Steps for Everybody*. Pacific Palisades, CA: The 12 Steps for Everybody, 2007.

May, Michelle. *Eat What You Love, Love What You Eat*. Austin, TX: Greenleaf Book Group Press, 2010.

McTaggart, Lynne. *The Bond: Connecting Through the Space Between Us*. New York: Free Press, 2011.

Miller, Alice. *For Your Own Good: Hidden Cruelty in Child-Rearing and the Roots of Violence*. 3rd ed. New York: Noonday Press, 1990.

Miller, Caroline Adams. *Feeding the Soul: Daily Meditations for Recovering from Eating Disorders*. New York: Bantam Books, 1991.

Myss, Caroline M. *Anatomy of the Spirit: The Seven Stages of Power and Healing*. New York: Three Rivers Press, 1996.

Naparstek, Belleruth. *Staying Well with Guided Imagery*. New York: Grand Central Publishing, 1994.

Orbach, Susie. *Fat is a Feminist Issue: The Anti-Diet Guide to Permanent Weight Loss*. New York: Paddington Press, 1978.

Overeaters Anonymous. Torrance, CA: Overeaters Anonymous, Inc., 1980.

Poppink, Joanna. *Healing Your Hungry Heart: Recovering from Your Eating Disorder*. San Francisco, CA: Conari Press, 2011.

Redfield, James. *The Celestine Prophecy: An Adventure*. New York: Warner Books, 1993.

Remen, Rachel Naomi. "On Defining Spirit," *IONS—Noetic Sciences Review*, 47:64 (Winter 1998).

Ross, Carolyn Coker. *The Binge Eating & Compulsive Overeating Workbook: An Integrated Approach to Overcoming Disordered Eating*. Oakland, CA: New Harbinger Publications, 2009.

Roth, Geneen. *Feeding the Hungry Heart: The Experience of Compulsive Eating.* Indianapolis, IN: Bobbs-Merrill, 1982.

———. *Women, Food and God: An Unexpected Path to Almost Everything.* New York: Scribner, 2010.

Sacker, Ira. *Regaining Your Self: Understanding and Conquering the Eating Disorder Identity.* Deerfield Beach, FL: Health Communications, 2007.

Schaef, Anne Wilson. *Women's Reality: An Emerging Female System in a White Male Society.* San Francisco, CA: HarperSanFrancisco, 1992.

Subby, Robert. *Lost in the Shuffle: The Co-Dependent Reality.* Deerfield Beach, FL: Health Communications, 1987.

Twelve Steps and Twelve Traditions. New York: Alcoholics Anonymous Pub., 1953.

The Twelve Steps and Twelve Traditions of Overeaters Anonymous. Torrance, CA: Overeaters Anonymous, 1993.

Virtue, Doreen. *Constant Craving: What Your Food Cravings Mean and How to Overcome Them.* Carlsbad, CA: Hay House, 1995.

Vitale, Joe, and Ihaleakala Hew Len. *Zero Limits: The Secret Hawaiian System for Wealth, Health, Peace, and More.* New York: John Wiley & Sons, 2008.

Whitfield, Charles. *Healing the Child Within.* Deerfield Beach, FL: Health Communications, 2006.

Williamson, Marianne. *A Woman's Worth.* New York: Ballantine, 1993.

———. *A Course in Weight Loss: 21 Spiritual Lessons for Surrendering Your Weight Forever.* Carlsbad, CA: Hay House, 2010.

Index

· · · · · ·

EFT (Emotional Freedom
Techniques), 83–90, **89**, 124, 126,
195; directions for, 87–89; and
Gary Craig, xiv, 80, 95; and RITT,
91, 105, 125, 126, 171, 195–96.
See also tapping techniques
EMDR (Eye Movement
Desensitization and Reprocessing):
and Francine Shapiro, 80
Emmons, Robert, 173
emotional eaters. *See* compulsive
overeaters
Emotional Freedom Techniques. *See*
EFT
empathy, 39, 108; and Nurturing
Parent, 117, 122, 125, 150, 171,
self-, 40, 123, 126, 164 and inner
emptiness, xvi, 3, 11, 30, 48, 123
energizers, 102, 105–106, 109, 196;
energy pick-me-ups, 106–107;
gratitude, 174, 178; meditation,
70. *See also* Sending Energy
Exercise
energy: defined, 79–80; personal
energy work, 99–109, 196; from
Source, 101–102
energy drains, 101, 105, 106, 107,
108–109, 196; criticism, 34–35,
133; drama, 108; feelings, 106,
108; low-energy people, 101,
103–105; victim mode, 43, 174,
177
energy medicine. *See* energy
psychology
energy level, monitoring, 109, 178,
184; affects of food, 187, 198–99;
identifying energizers and drains,
105, 109, 196
energy psychology, 79, 98, 108–109,
124–25, 167; description, xviii,
80, 81. *See also* EFT; RITT; tapping
techniques
energy tests, 185–186, 187, 198. *See
also* muscle tests
Epstein, Gerald, 72
Eye Movement Desensitization and
Reprocessing. *See* EMDR

fast food, xvi, 17, 183, 199, 202
Father Knows Best, 2

feelings: eased with tapping, xviii,
82, 85, 90, 98–99, 108–109;
expressing, 30, 76, 106, 175;
facing, 12, 26, 35, 47, 114; guilt
and shame, 8, 137, 138, 140,
144; journaling, 26, 33, 192; list
of uncomfortable, 24–25; pushed
away with food, xv-xvi, 22, 23,
86, 90. *See also* anxieties
Feinstein, David, 124–25
fight-or-flight response, 81, 124
food: for comfort, 16, 48, 61; to
escape, xvii, 18, 90, 115; feeling
connection with, x, xvi, 22, 23,
86, 192; to fill inner emptiness, 3,
4, 11, 28, 123; as a pick-me-up,
99, 105; as a drug, 12, 17–18,
48–49, 113, 160
food-mood diary, 22–25, 26, 33, 89,
192
Food obsession, aleviating with:
amends, 152, 157; inner work, 138,
147, 159, 207–208; psychotherapy,
46; reframe, 175; spirituality, 54,
194; tapping, 99, 196
Ford, Debbie, 111
forgiveness, 160–71, 198; requesting,
154, 157; in RITT, 94, 98; self-,
40, 150, 161, 163–64, 171
Fourth-Step inventory, 36, 140–45,
147, 149

Gawain, Shakti, 72, 74
Gilbert, Susan K., 210
God. *See* Higher Power
gratitude, 172–74, 198, 210; as an
energizer, 105, 178; list, 173, 178,
198, 203; prayers, 65, 70, 179;
reframe, 174–77; research project
173

habits: around food, 99, 182–183,
201; developing new, 30, 45, 109,
199
H.A.L.T. (hungry, angry, lonely, tired),
184, 198–99
Hammarskjöld, Dag, 15
Haskvitz, Sylvia, 180
have to: changed to *choose to*, 42, 43,
45, 46, 194

Hay, Louise, 43
Healthy Adult: described, 118; conversing with Inner Child, 121–24, 126, 196; dialogue with Inner Critic, 129–36; need for, 117, 118–19; nonjudgmental, 122, 125, 146, 147, 150; dialogue with sad part, 165–67, 171. *See also* Right-Hand/Left-Hand Dialogue
Hew Len, Dr. Ihaleakala, 196. *See also* Ho'oponopono
Higher Power, 55–61, 70, 146–47, 194; letter to, 58–59, 61; as a Loving Presence, 57–58, 61, 65, 149; parts work with, 135, 166–67; in RITT, 92–96, 168; and Twelve-Step recovery, 36–37, 64. *See also* prayer and meditation
Ho'oponopono, 169–171, 198; cleaning, 170
"How Heavy is Your Bag?," 162–163
hunger: emotional, xvi, 10, 31, 109; identifying, 179, 180, 183, 187; mouth, 183; lack of physical, 3, 15–16, 22; spiritual, 31, 51
Huxley, Aldous, xx

Inner Child, 12, 114–26, 137, 196, 201; described, 115, 116; and tapping, 124–25. *See also* Right-Hand/Left-Hand Dialogue
Inner Child guided imagery, 119–121
Inner Critic, 12, 127–36, 197; blaming and shaming, 34, 128, 130–33, 164; described, 127. *See also* Chair Work; Two Hands Talking
Inner-Work Walks, 205–206
Irving, Washington, 211

John-Roger, 53–54
journaling: health benefits, 27, 173; as a self-help tool, 12, 26–31, 106, 114, 192, 200, 201
journey: healing, ix, 37, inward, 15, 34, 48, 159, 208; of recovery, xi, xvii, 43, 193, 207; to wholeness, 111, 117

Katie, Byron, 193

Lean Test, 185–186
Leave it to Beaver, 2
Loving Presence. *See* Higher Power
love: from families, xii–xiii, 13, 114; using food for, 7, 9; from Healthy Adult, 122, 129, 130, 132–33, 135; for Inner Child, 116, 120, 123–24; self-, 147, 160; unconditional, 57–58, 59, 61, 117, 149
low energy. *See* energy drains
Luccock, H. E., 33

Masci, Robin Trainor, xiii, 91, 102, 167–68, 169
May, Michelle, 179–180
McCullough, Michael, 173
McTaggart, Lynne, 40
meditations, 65–70, 72, 77, 164; aspects of, 65–66; Conscious Breathing Meditation, 66–67; gazing, 68–70; for stress management, 70, 105; Walking Meditation, 68. *See also* prayer and meditation
meridian therapies. *See* energy psychology; tapping techniques
Miller, Alice, 112
mini inventory, 140–45, 160, 197; giving it away, 146–51, making amends, 151–52, 156
Miyazawa, Kenji, 209
Morrissey, Mary Manin, 167, 171
muscle tests, 82–84. *See also* energy tests
Myss, Caroline, 161

Naparstek, Belleruth, 72
Niebuhr, Reinhold. *See* Serenity Prayer
Nonviolent communication. *See* NVC
Nurturing Parent. *See* Healthy Adult
NVC (Nonviolent Communication) 39–40, 180

obesity; x, xv, 13, 15
Oprah, 168
orthorexia nervosa: and Steve Bratman, 181
Overeaters Anonymous (OA), xviii, 37, 138
Oz, Dr., 79

pain, emotional, xvi, 3, 9, 17–18, 23,
48; released with tapping, 80, 82,
83, 85, 99, 108–109
parts work, 127–36, 171, 197. *See
also* Chair Work; Right-Hand/
Left-Hand Dialogue; Two Hands
Talking
personal growth, xvii, 30, 48, 208;
Inner-Work Walks, 205–206; self-
awareness, 14, 17, 27, 111, 192;
self-empowerment, 43, 46, 167,
177, 194; transformation, xx, 34,
121, 208
Powell, Chris, xvi
prayer, 62–65, 70, 173, 179;
children's 62; and meditation, 37,
51, 62, 194; types of, 65
Prayer: Lord's, 62–63; Serenity, 63;
Seventh Step, 64; Shema, 63;
Third Step, 64
"Pretender, The Great," 6
Proust, Marcel, xii
psychotherapy, xvii, 13, 27–28,
46–49, 194

Rapidly Integrated Transformation
Technique. *See* RITT
Redfern, Suzanne, 210
Reframe, 179, 198; examples of,
174–77
Remen, Rachel Naomi, 52–53
resentment, 161, 167; and
compulsive eating, 160, 161–162;
letting go of, 105, 170, 171;
listed in Fourth-Step inventory,
141–42
"Richard Cory," 9
Right-Hand/Left-Hand Dialogue,
121–26, 136, 196–97, 201. *See
also* parts work
RITT (Rapidly Integrated
Transformation Technique),
91–99, **92**, 168, 195–96; for
cravings, 95–99; directions,
92–94. *See also* EFT and RITT
Rosenberg, Marshall. *See* NVC
Roth, Geneen, 180
Rust, Jeanne, xi, xiv, 180

TAB (Touch and Breathe): and John
Diepold, 81, 91
Tapas Acupressure Technique. *See* TAT
Tapping techniques, 82, 105, 106,
184, 192; why they work, 81–82,
124–25; experiences with, 84–86,
98–99, 168. *See also* EFT; energy
psychology; RITT; TFT
TAT (Tapas Acupressure Technique):
and Tapas Fleming, 80
TFT (Thought Field Therapy): and
Roger Callahan, 82–83
Therapy. *See* psychotherapy
Third Step Prayer, 64
Thought Field Therapy. *See* TFT
Touch and Breathe. *See* TAB
traumas, 112–113; compared to
splinters, 111–12, 114; healing,
81–82, 117, 124–25, 167–68
triggers, 13, 115–16; identifying, 26,
144, 181–84, 187; list of, 129,
199–203. *See also* sabotage
Twelve-Step Recovery, xvii, 35;
Promises of, 159–160; and self-
discovery, 13, 115, 140, 206–207;
spirituality, 12, 36–37, 57, 91;
support groups, xviii, 37–38, 114
Two Hands Talking, 129, 133, 136,
197. *See also* parts work

Velveteen Rabbit, The: being real,
139–140
vision boards, 75–76, 77, 195
visualizations, creative, xviii, 71–75,
76–77; 195, 201; pink bubble, 74,
75, 77; Weight Loss Visualization,
73–74
Vitale, Joe, 169–170

walking, 44, 61, 64, 105. *See also*
Inner-Work Walks
WHEE (Whole Health Easily and
Effectively): and Daniel Benor, 81,
204; directions, 204–205
Whitfield, Charles, 115
Woolf, Virginia, 137

Ziggy, 34

About the Author

....

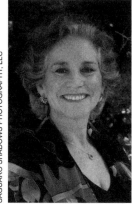

MERYL HERSHEY BECK is a therapist (Licensed Professional Clinical Counselor) with a longtime personal and professional relationship to the recovery movement. She is trained in EMDR, energy medicine, and other healing modalities. She is also a member of a number of national and international organizations working with eating disorders.

Meryl spent the first half of her life as a closet eater, gaining weight and feeling overwrought. Once she became active in Twelve-Step support groups, the bingeing started to wane. Intent on uncovering the root cause of her overeating, Meryl began to incorporate new approaches in her quest for self-understanding. As a counselor, teacher, and author, Meryl joyfully shares these many tools and techniques that skyrocket personal growth and alleviate emotional eating.

She lives in Tucson, Arizona. Visit her at *energizedforlife .com*.

To Our Readers